# Eosinophilic Esophagitis

*Editor*

DAVID A. KATZKA

## GASTROINTESTINAL ENDOSCOPY CLINICS OF NORTH AMERICA

www.giendo.theclinics.com

*Consulting Editor*
CHARLES J. LIGHTDALE

January 2018 • Volume 28 • Number 1

**ELSEVIER**

1600 John F. Kennedy Boulevard • Suite 1800 • Philadelphia, Pennsylvania, 19103-2899

http://www.theclinics.com

**GASTROINTESTINAL ENDOSCOPY CLINICS OF NORTH AMERICA Volume 28, Number 1**
**January 2018 ISSN 1052-5157, ISBN-13: 978-0-323-56639-1**

Editor: Kerry Holland
Developmental Editor: Donald Mumford

*Gastrointestinal Endoscopy Clinics of North America* (ISSN 1052-5157) is published quarterly by Elsevier Inc., 360 Park Avenue South, New York, NY 10010-1710. Months of issue are January, April, July, and October. Business and Editorial Offices: 1600 John F. Kennedy Blvd., Suite 1800, Philadelphia, PA, 19103-2899. Periodicals postage paid at New York, NY and additional mailing offices. Subscription prices are $349.00 per year for US individuals, $593.00 per year for US institutions, $100.00 per year for US students and residents, $385.00 per year for Canadian individuals, $702.00 per year for Canadian institutions, $474.00 per year for international individuals, $702.00 per year for international institutions, and $245.00 per year for Canadian and foreign students/residents. To receive student/resident rate, orders must be accompanied by name of affiliated institution, date of term, and the *signature* of program/residency coordinator on institution letterhead. Orders will be billed at individual rate until proof of status is received. Foreign air speed delivery is included in all *Clinics* subscription prices. All prices are subject to change without notice. **POSTMASTER:** Send address change to *Gastrointestinal Endoscopy Clinics of North America*, Elsevier Health Sciences Division, Subscription Customer Service, 3251 Riverport Lane, Maryland Heights, MO 63043. **Customer Service: 1-800-654-2452 (US). From outside the United States, call 1-314-447-8871. Fax: 1-314-447-8029. E-mail: JournalsCustomerService-usa@elsevier.com (for print support) or JournalsOnlineSupport-usa@elsevier.com (for online support)**.

*Reprints.* For copies of 100 or more, of articles in this publication, please contact the Commercial Reprints Department, Elsevier Inc., 360 Park Avenue South, New York, NY 10010-1710. Tel. 212-633-3874; Fax: 212-633-3820; E-mail: reprints@elsevier.com.

*Gastrointestinal Endoscopy Clinics of North America* is covered in *Excerpta Medica, MEDLINE/PubMed (Index Medicus), and MEDLINE/MEDLARS.*

# Contributors

## CONSULTING EDITOR

**CHARLES J. LIGHTDALE, MD**
Professor of Medicine, Division of Digestive and Liver Diseases, Columbia University Medical Center, New York, New York, USA

## EDITOR

**DAVID A. KATZKA, MD**
Professor and Consultant in Medicine, Department of Gastroenterology, Mayo Clinic, Rochester, Minnesota, USA

## AUTHORS

**JEFFREY A. ALEXANDER, MD, FACP**
Associate Professor of Medicine, Division of Gastroenterology and Hepatology, Mayo Clinic School of Medicine, Rochester, Minnesota, USA

**FREDERIC CLAYTON, MD**
Professor, Department of Pathology, The University of Utah, Huntsman Cancer Institute, Salt Lake City, Utah, USA

**STEVEN B. CLAYTON, MD, FAAFP, FACP**
Gastroenterology and Liver Center, Greenville Health System, Clinical Assistant Professor of Medicine, University of South Carolina School of Medicine–Greenville, Greenville, South Carolina, USA

**NIRMALA GONSALVES, MD**
Associate Professor of Medicine, Division of Gastroenterology and Hepatology, Northwestern University Feinberg School of Medicine, Chicago, Illinois, USA

**IKUO HIRANO, MD**
Professor of Medicine, Division of Gastroenterology, Northwestern University Feinberg School of Medicine, Chicago, Illinois, USA

**ROBERT T. KAVITT, MD, MPH**
Assistant Professor of Medicine, Director, Center for Esophageal Diseases, Section of Gastroenterology, Hepatology, and Nutrition, The University of Chicago Medicine, Chicago, Illinois, USA

**ANNA MARIA LIPOWSKA, MD**
Gastroenterology Fellow, Section of Gastroenterology, Hepatology, and Nutrition, The University of Chicago Medicine, Chicago, Illinois, USA

**JONATHAN E. MARKOWITZ, MD, MSCE**
Chief, Pediatric Gastroenterology and Nutrition, Children's Hospital Greenville
Health System, Professor of Pediatrics, University of South Carolina School of
Medicine–Greenville, Greenville, South Carolina, USA

**FOUAD J. MOAWAD, MD**
Associate Professor of Medicine, Division of Gastroenterology, Scripps Clinic, Anderson
Medical Pavilion, La Jolla, California, USA

**KATHRYN PETERSON, MD, MSci**
Associate Professor of Medicine, Division of Gastroenterology, The University of Utah,
Salt Lake City, Utah, USA

**JOEL E. RICHTER, MD, MACG, FACP**
Professor of Medicine, Hugh F. Culverhouse Chair for Esophageal Disorders, Director,
Division of Digestive Diseases & Nutrition, Director, Joy McCann Culverhouse Center for
Swallowing Disorders, University of South Florida Morsani College of Medicine, Tampa,
Florida, USA

**EKATERINA SAFRONEEVA, PhD**
Institute of Social and Preventive Medicine, University of Bern, Bern, Switzerland

**ALAIN M. SCHOEPFER, MD**
Division of Gastroenterology and Hepatology, Centre Hospitalier Universitaire Vaudois
(CHUV), Lausanne, Switzerland

**ALEX STRAUMANN, MD**
Swiss EoE Clinic, Olten, Switzerland; Division of Gastroenterology and Hepatology,
University Hospital Zurich, Zurich, Switzerland

# Contents

Eosinophilic esophagitis is an adaptive immune response to patient-specific antigens, mostly foods. Eosinophilic esophagitis is not solely immunoglobulin E–mediated and is likely characterized by Th2 lymphocytes with an impaired esophageal barrier function. The key cytokines and chemokines are thymic stromal lymphopoeitin, interleukin-13, CCL26/eotaxin-3, and transforming growth factor-β, all involved in eosinophil recruitment and remodeling. Chronic food dysphagia and food impactions, the feared late complications, are related in part to dense subepithelial fibrosis, likely induced by interleukin-13 and transforming growth factor-β.

Eosinophilic esophagitis (EoE) is a rapidly emerging allergy-mediated condition encountered frequently in clinical practice. It presents with failure to thrive, nausea, and vomiting in children and is a common reason for dysphagia and food impaction in adults. Several institution-based and population-based studies have reported the frequency of EoE over the past few years. The incidence and prevalence of EoE vary depending on the method of data collection. In population-based studies using national registries, the incidence appears to be increasing, currently estimated to be approximately 10 cases/100,000 persons annually, whereas the prevalence is reported between 10 and 57 cases/100,000 persons.

Eosinophilic esophagitis (EoE) is an increasingly prevalent chronic condition characterized by eosinophilic infiltration of the esophageal epithelium accompanied by esophageal symptoms. The number of new diagnoses is growing worldwide in both pediatric and adult populations. Differences in disease distribution and presentation have been found, varying by gender, race, and other characteristics. This article examines the existing literature and provides insight into the demographic features of EoE.

EoE include proton pump inhibitors and swallowed topical steroids. Several biologic therapies are currently under evaluation and some of them have shown promising results in improving biologic endpoints and patient-reported outcomes.

Eosinophilic esophagitis is characterized by dense mucosal eosinophilia with symptoms of esophageal dysfunction. Because the incidence and prevalence are increasing, understanding the available treatments is imperative. This article highlights evolution and advancements in dietary treatment, supports the notion that food antigens drive this disease, and discusses the advantages, limitations, and future of dietary therapy. Medical and dietary therapies are effective treatments and the optimal approach should be individualized based on patient goals and available local resources. Dietary therapy has been effective, and further studies will help identify optimal approaches to dietary therapy.

In eosinophilic esophagitis, the main cause of solid-food dysphagia is tissue remodeling resulting in strictures and narrowed esophagus. Endoscopy and biopsies help to identify the degree of inflammation but often miss the fibrosis. Although initially considered dangerous, esophageal dilation has evolved into an extremely effective and safe treatment in fibrostenotic disease. The key is starting low with small-diameter bougies or balloons, and gradually dilating the esophagus and strictures to 16 to 18 mm. Results in more than 1000 adults and children have shown low rates of complications, especially perforations, and no deaths, but postprocedure chest pain is common.

Eosinophilic esophagitis advances parallel the increased prevalence. Developments include refining the diagnostic criteria, identifying risk factors, appreciating the contribution of inflammatory pathways, recognizing the importance of subepithelial remodeling, validating trial endpoints, defining a role for biological therapies, and optimizing dietary therapy. Endoscopic outcomes have emerged as endpoints in trials of novel therapeutics. Expanding efforts seek to develop less-invasive methods to assess disease activity, thereby reducing the burden of repeated endoscopic procedures during elimination diets. The functional lumen imaging probe is now identified as a determinant of complications with potential utility as a therapeutic endpoint.

# GASTROINTESTINAL ENDOSCOPY CLINICS OF NORTH AMERICA

---

**RELATED INTEREST**

*Gastroenterology Clinics of North America,* June 2014, (Vol. 43, No. 2)
**Eosinophilic Esophagitis**
Ikuo Hirano, *Editor*

---

**THE CLINICS ARE AVAILABLE ONLINE!**
Access your subscription at:
www.theclinics.com

# Foreword

# Eosinophilic Esophagitis: New Insights and Management

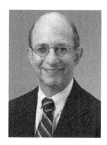

Charles J. Lightdale, MD
*Consulting Editor*

It is notable that 10 years have flown by since the last issue of *Gastrointestinal Endoscopy Clinics of North America* devoted to eosinophilic esophagitis (EoE). It was clear to me that the time had certainly come for another such issue. During this past decade, there has been remarkable progress in our understanding of this complex allergic disease. As the incidence of EoE continues to increase in children and adults, clinicians have become much more aware of its acute and chronic manifestations and significantly more concerned about accurate diagnosis and the most effective treatment approaches.

Like many first-year medical students, I remember being instantly fascinated with eosinophils on doing my first microscopic exams of blood smears. These white blood cells are granulocytes that are eosinophilic, showing up a striking brick-red when stained with the acid dye eosin. No eosinophils are seen in the normal esophagus, but frequently appear in inflammatory and allergic conditions. Eosinophilic disease can occur throughout the gastrointestinal tract, but it is the esophagus that has become the most important organ with its increasing incidence. I feel very fortunate to have, as editor for this issue of the *Gastrointestinal Endoscopy Clinics of North America*, Dr David A. Katzka, a widely recognized expert in esophageal diseases, and a world leader in the field of EoE.

Dr Katzka has marshaled an all-star list of authors to produce a comprehensive state-of-the-art review. The first article on pathophysiology and definition is critical. Much of the recent progress in the field reflects a deepening understanding of the biologic processes fundamental to EoE, which will almost certainly lead to further gains in management. Eosinophilic esophagitis is abbreviated as EoE to differentiate it from erosive esophagitis (EE) related to gastroesophageal reflux disease (GERD), yet the relationship of EoE to GERD remains problematic in some cases, and both may exist simultaneously. The existence of esophageal eosinophilia with symptoms responsive

Gastrointest Endoscopy Clin N Am 28 (2018) ix–x
https://doi.org/10.1016/j.giec.2017.10.002
1052-5157/18/© 2017 Published by Elsevier Inc.

to proton pump inhibitors (PPI-responsive EoE) seems to represent an important subset. In this regard, other articles deal with the epidemiology of EoE, the relationship of symptoms to biologic findings, and diagnosis by endoscopy, biopsy, and radiology. Various manifestations of the disease in children and adults are also reviewed, and important new scoring systems useful in management are presented. Therapy is thoroughly covered in three articles unitized according to pharmacology approaches, dietary management, and endoscopic treatments mostly focused on fixed strictures and stenosis. As presented in the final article relating to the future, with the rapid pace of continued laboratory discoveries, better precision-based treatments seem likely before long. This is an issue that should appeal to specialists in esophageal diseases, and to most clinical gastroenterologists in both adult and pediatric practice. It's a great read, packed with scientific and practical information. Don't miss it.

Charles J. Lightdale, MD
Department of Medicine
Columbia University Medical Center
161 Fort Washington Avenue
New York, NY 10032, USA

*E-mail address:*
CJL18@columbia.edu

# Preface
# Eosinophilic Esophagitis

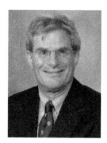

David A. Katzka, MD
*Editor*

The research and knowledge base of eosinophilic esophagitis continues to expand at remarkable speed. As a result, the spectrum of clinical manifestations and treatments changes at a pace that mandates frequent updates on this fascinating disease. In this issue of *Gastrointestinal Endoscopy Clinics of North America*, we summarize all the latest literature on eosinophilic esophagitis. For example, interest in eosinophilic esophagitis by the basic scientists has spawned a far greater insight into the cellular and molecular pathogenesis of the disease. In diagnosis and treatment, the field is shifting toward the use of validated scoring systems not only for research but also for clinical monitoring of the disease. Finally, future directions are predicted, though with the rate of change we are finding with eosinophilic esophagitis, this work may all be accomplished by the time it is needed to write another issue on this topic!

This issue is dedicated to my loves, Margie, Emma, and Will.

David A. Katzka, MD
Department of Gastroenterology
Mayo Clinic
200 First Avenue, SW
Rochester, MN 55905, USA

*E-mail address:*
Katzka.David@mayo.edu

Gastrointest Endoscopy Clin N Am 28 (2018) xi
https://doi.org/10.1016/j.giec.2017.10.001
1052-5157/18/© 2017 Published by Elsevier Inc.

# Eosinophilic Esophagitis
## Pathophysiology and Definition

 CrossMark

Frederic Clayton, MD[a], Kathryn Peterson, MD, MSci[b],*

## KEYWORDS

- Eosinophilic esophagitis • Pathophysiology • PPI-REE
- Proton pump inhibitor responsive esophageal eosinophilia

## KEY POINTS

- Eosinophilic esophagitis is an atopic, inflammatory condition of the esophagus characterized by eosinophlic infiltrate with subsequent fibrosis and reduced quality of life.
- Both genetics and the environment contribute to disease with risk identified in distant relatives, and external factors compound one's risk for disease.
- The pathophysiology results from complex interplay of many allergic and inflammatory cells including eosinophils, mast cells, basophils, and lymphocytes.
- Dense subepithelial fibrosis, mediated by TGF-β and associated cytokines, is a common complication of the disease.

## OVERVIEW

Eosinophilic esophagitis (EoE) is an adaptive immune response to patient-specific antigens, mostly foods. EoE is not IgE-mediated and is instead likely mediated by Th2 lymphocytes (**Fig. 1**). The esophageal barrier function is impaired. The key cytokines and chemokines are thymic stromal lymphopoeitin (TSLP), interleukin (IL)-13, CCL26/eotaxin-3, and transforming growth factor-β1 (TGFB1). Chronic solid food dysphagia, the feared late complication, is caused by dense subepithelial fibrosis, likely induced by IL-13 and TGFB1.

## DEFINITION

The current consensus criteria needed to define EoE require esophageal symptoms, an esophageal biopsy with 15 or more eosinophils in at least one high-power field

Disclosure Statement: None of the authors have any relevant disclosures.
[a] Department of Pathology, The University of Utah, Huntsman Cancer Hospital, 1950 Circle of Hope, Room N3100, Salt Lake City, UT 84112, USA; [b] Division of Gastroenterology, The University of Utah, 30 North 1900 East SOM 4R118, Salt Lake City, UT 84132, USA
* Corresponding author.
*E-mail address:* Kathryn.peterson@hsc.utah.edu

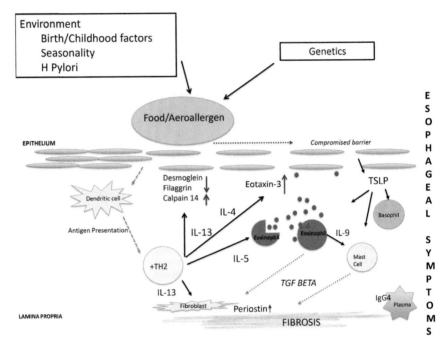

**Fig. 1.** The pathogenesis of EoE involves the complex interplay between genetics, a strong influence of environment, and antigenic stimuli from food or aeroallergens. The current paradigm suggests food and/or aeroallergen exposure with subsequent antigen presentation by dendritic cells and/or epithelium initiates disease. From antigen presentation, T cells are differentiated into Th2 cells secreting interleukin (IL)-4, IL-5, and IL-13. IL-4 and IL-13 are responsible for secretion of eotaxin-3 and upregulation of periostin in epithelial cells and fibroblasts. IL-13 has multiple effects including disruption of the epithelial barrier via actions on calpain, desmoglein, and filaggrin along with simulation of eosinophils. IL-5 is a key cytokine involved in eosinophil recruitment into the esophagus with a possible effect on mast cells. Eosinophils cytolyze releasing granule proteins toxic to epithelium. Eosinophils also release IL-9 aiding in proliferation and differentiation of mast cells. TSLP influences Th2 responses with specific influence on antigen presentation and basophil mobilization into esophageal tissue. TGF-β influences remodeling with subsequent fibrosis in the lamina propria. Plasma cells rich in IgG4 of unclear significance are found abundantly in the lamina propria. TGF, transforming growth factor; TSLP, thymic stromal lymphopoietin.

despite an 8-week or longer treatment with maximal dose proton pump inhibitor (PPI) therapy, and exclusion of other causes for esophageal eosinophilia (**Box 1**).[1]

Subsequent data challenge the exclusion of PPI-responsive patients from the definition of EoE; PPI-responsive patients can clinically and pathologically have essentially identical disease.[2] For example, the esophageal tissue transcriptomes are extremely similar.[3,4] In vitro studies show that PPIs directly block the IL-13/STAT6/eotaxin-3 signaling pathway, and, thus, response to PPI does not implicate acid reflux as causal to the disease.[5,6] PPI responders also respond to food elimination diets,[7] implying that the PPI responsive cases, like classically defined EoE, are induced by an aberrant food antigen–driven immune response. Clearly, PPI-responsive cases are extremely similar to EoE on a clinical and a molecular basis and probably should be considered together or as an extremely close disease variant.

> **Box 1**
> **Diseases associated with esophageal eosinophilia**
>
> Reflux esophagitis
>
> Eosinophilic gastroenteritis
>
> Celiac disease
>
> Crohn disease
>
> Infection
>
> Hypereosinophilic syndrome
>
> Achalasia
>
> Drug hypersensitivity
>
> Vasculitis and eosinophilic granulomatosis polyangiitis
>
> Connective tissue diseases
>
> Graft-versus-host disease

Other problems relate to the histologic counts. The size of the microscopic high-power field varies in different microscopes and thus calculation of eosinophil density per high-power field. A diagnosis based on a quantitative histologic criterion inevitably has borderline and false-negative cases. Pediatric patients with 5 to 14 eosinophils per high-power field are at risk of subsequently developing dysphagia and EoE.[8,9] Furthermore, tissue eosinophilia is patchy; multiple biopsies are needed for adequate tissue sampling.[10] Scoring systems with immunostaining or histologic criteria other than eosinophil counts have been proposed, but are not widely used.[9,11]

## CLINICAL SYMPTOMS

The definition of EoE requires esophageal dysfunction. Symptoms vary by patient age and gender. They can manifest as nausea, food aversion, and failure to thrive in children versus swallowing difficulty, food impactions, and refractory heartburn in adults.[12] The main chronic symptom is dysphagia, particularly of solid foods, often with food impaction. The dysphagia can be disabling leading to significantly reduced quality of life.[13,14] In fact, EoE is the most common cause of food impactions in young adults.[15] Female patients are more likely than men to present with chest pain or heartburn rather than dysphagia.[16] Unfortunately, symptoms correlate poorly with the extent of esophageal eosinophilia and histologic response to therapy particularly in the presence of fibrotic strictures.[17,18] As a result, the definition of EoE is expanding to include measures of symptom response in addition to tissue eosinophilia.

## PATHOPHYSIOLOGY
### Genetic Insights

Different approaches have been taken to identify EoE-associated genes, including candidate gene studies, and genome-wide association studies (GWAS) and phenome-wide association studies. Early candidate gene analyses identified genetic variants at CCL 26 (eotaxin 3), FLG (filaggrin), CRLF2, and DSG1 (desmoglein 1) as possible associated genes (**Table 1**). The first GWAS performed identified risk variants at locus 5q22, which holds the gene for TSLP, a gene commonly found in atopic

**Table 1**
**Common gene associations with susceptibility of eosinophilic esophagitis**

| Gene | Identification | Proposed Function |
|------|---------------|-------------------|
| Eotaxin-3 | Single gene association | Chemotaxis for eosinophils and basophils |
| Filaggrin | Single gene association | Epidermal barrier–associated with eczema risk |
| TGFB1 | Singe gene association | Wound repair and remodeling |
| TSLP | Genome-wide association | Released in response to epithelial damage Associated with atopy and activation of Th2 responses |
| LRRC32 | Genome-wide association | Controls TGF-β from T regulatory cells |
| ANKRD27 | Genome-wide association | Trafficking of melanogenic enzymes |
| C11orf30 | Genome-wide association | Increases risk for sensitization |
| Calpain14 | Genome-wide association | Esophageal-specific, calcium-activated protease with ability to affect esophageal barrier function |
| STAT6 | Genome-wide association | Activated by IL-4/IL-13 Drives expression of many genes in EoE |

disease. TSLP is expressed in the esophageal epithelium in EoE and has the ability to influence different immune responses in allergy.[19]

Prior GWAS identified variants at CPN14, LRRC32/C11orf30, STAT6, TSLP/WDR36, and ANKRD27.[20] Additionally, PheWas (phenotypic association studies where a set of candidate genome-wide genetic variants were assessed along with a range of phenotypes) found EoE associations with PTEN, TGFBR1/TGFBR2/PBN, and IL-5/IL-13. IL-5/IL-13 variants have been associated with comorbid eosinophilia as often seen in EoE.[21] Many of the risk loci found are associated with allergic sensitization, atopic dermatitis, allergic rhinitis, and asthma, which are often seen concurrently with EoE. As a result, it is difficult to specifically attach these abnormalities to EoE as opposed to a more generalized atopic phenotype. TSLP affects many cells and primes a Th2 response in multiple different cell lines, most importantly epithelial and hematopoietic. LRRC32 plays a role in surface expression and signaling of TGF-β signaling in T regulatory functions.[22] C11orf30 has been shown to increase one's risk for polysensitization to allergens.[23] STAT6 is the transcription factor activated by IL-4/IL-13 and facilitates the expression of many genes in the EoE transcriptome.[24,25] CAPN14 (calpain 14), a calcium activated intracellular protease expressed exclusively in the esophagus, is upregulated in EoE.[26] CAPN14, induced by IL-13,[27] regulates DSG1 (desmoglein-1), thus disrupting the epithelial barrier.[28] LRRC31 regulates kallikreins, also disrupting the epithelial barrier function effects.[29]

A twin study examined the concurrence of disease in monozygotic versus dizygotic twins and emphasized the importance of environment in the pathogenesis of EoE.[30] A recent family study found increased risk for developing EoE even in distant family members.[31] These family studies emphasize the importance of environment in addition to genetics in the pathogenesis of EoE.

## EPIDEMIOLOGY AND ENVIRONMENT

Clues to the pathophysiology of EoE come from epidemiologic studies. EoE is considered an atopic disease; most patients with EoE have concurrent atopic diseases including asthma, eczema, or seasonal rhinitis.[32] Other environmental studies have elucidated much about the disease.[33,34] EoE is usually driven by food antigens.

In children up to 95% respond to elemental diet with reduction of tissue eosinophilia.[34,35] Adult data are less robust (likely from reduced compliance), but greater than 70% of adults respond to an elemental diet.[36,37] Aeroallergens may also contribute to disease.[38,39]

Early life factors are associated with altered EoE risk, including breastfeeding and penicillin allergy. Early antibiotic use, presumably by altering the intestinal microbiome, increases the EoE risk six-fold.[40–42]

EoE is about 2:1 male-predominant.[43] Rural lifestyles may lead to increased incidence of EoE.[44] *Helicobacter pylori* infection may protect against the disease.[45,46] Seasonal variations in detection of disease are disputed.[47] Typical adult symptoms are dysphagia and chest pain, whereas in children symptoms often are vague, such as feeding difficulties, nausea, failure to thrive, and abdominal pain often reported.[12] Symptoms only modestly correlate with disease activity.[17] In children, the lack of uniform symptoms contributes to the difficulty assessing symptom correlation to disease activity.

## *Epithelial Pathobiology*

The epithelium plays pivotal roles in the development of EoE by inducing crucial signals through cytokines, such as eotaxin-3. The epithelium also has reduced transepithelial resistance and impedance, implying increased permeability and antigen exposure.[37,48–50] In fact, baseline impedance (throughout the esophagus) may be impaired.[51] Alterations in expression of desmoglein-1, calpain 14, and LRRC31 induce loss of epithelial barrier function. Oncostatin M overexpression in EoE also reduces transepithelial esophageal resistance and contributes to the spongiosis (histologic appearance of dilated intercellular spaces) typical of EoE.[52]

Microarray and reverse transcriptase polymerase chain reaction studies identified increased expression of ALOX15 and tumor necrosis factor-α–induced factor 6 (TNFAIP6) and underexpression of FLG, SLURP1, and cysteine-rich secretory protein 3 (CRISP3) in EoE.[53] Immunohistochemistry for FLG found no FLG in active EoE biopsies, but FLG expression was regained after treatment.

## EOSINOPHILS

The hallmark of EoE is presence of at least 15 eosinophils per high-power field. Eotaxin-3, the major EoE chemokine for eosinophil chemotaxis, is markedly upregulated in EoE biopsies.[54] The distribution of eosinophils is patchy; multiple biopsies are needed to reliably identify disease.[55] Eosinophils are activated in the esophagus in EoE; degranulation and cytolysis are common.[56,57] Levels of granule proteins in disease are increased and are often found in areas with few or no intact eosinophils.[58–60] Eosinophils also can secrete T-cell-activating cytokines and can serve as antigen-presenting cells with major histocompatibility cell-II presentation.[61] Eosinophils release TGFB1, IL-5, IL-13, RANTES, PAF, and LTC4. Eosinophil major basic protein increases esophageal expression of FGF9 in EoE. FGF9 serves to aid in activation of fibroblasts.[62]

## T CELLS

In EoE, the esophageal population of CD3+, CD4+, and CD8+ T cells are all increased in the esophageal mucosa.[63] In many immune responses, CD4+ T cells are activated via antigen-presenting cells. In allergic responses, the classic T cells involved are Th2 cells. Murine models suggest increased levels of Th2 cells in esophageal tissues of EoE. Absence of CD4+ T cells protects mice from the stimulation of eosinophilic esophageal infiltration, whereas ablation of CD8[+] cells or B cells does not affect disease status, implicating Th2 cells as the key cell type inducing the antigen-specific adaptive immune response in EoE.[64] IL-13- and IL-5-producing Th2 cells, characteristically also expressing CD161 and hematopoietic prostaglandin D synthase, were recently detected in human EoE and other eosinophilic gastrointestinal disorders and atopic dermatitis.[65]

## REGULATORY T CELLS

Regulatory T cells are increased in esophageal biopsies in content per unit area or volume,[66] but are not increased as a proportion of total T cells.[67] Without knowing whether the regulatory T cells are activated in EoE, their significance is unclear.

## INNATE NATURAL KILLER T CELLS AND TYPE 2 INNATE LYMPHOID

Innate natural killer T cells have been studied in mouse models and in pediatric human patients with EoE. Innate natural killer T cells are a subset of lymphocytes that produce Th2 cytokines, particularly IL-13, and are implicated in the pathogenesis of Th2 mediated responses.[68–71] Type 2 innate lymphocyte 2 cells will express CRTH2 activating TH2 responses and have been identified in tissues of ptitents with EoE.

## MAST CELLS

Esophageal mast cell content is increased in EoE.[72] Microarray analysis of EoE tissues shows upregulation of many mast cell–associated genes.[73] Others have postulated an association of mast cells with TGF-$\beta$, the process of remodeling, effects on smooth muscle function, and symptom generation. The increased tissue mast cell content lessens in response to food elimination diets and topical corticosteroids.[74,75] Murine models suggest that mast cell numbers increase in parallel with eosinophils with EoE activity. Mast cells have little or no influence on promoting esophageal eosinophilia but do cause smooth muscle hypertrophy.[76] In a murine model, eosinophil-derived IL-9 increases mast cell tissue content and activation. IL-5 may contribute to increased mast cells in the esophagus of EoE directly or indirectly.[77] Trials of antibodies to IL-5 have demonstrated a decrease in eosinophils and mast cells.[78]

## BASOPHILS

Basophils can initiate and maintain an allergic response. Increased esophageal basophilia is found in EoE.[31] Noti and colleagues[79] suggest that basophils are critical to eosinophil recruitment in a murine model of EoE via TSLP.

## MAIN CHEMOKINES/CYTOKINES
### Interleukin-13

IL-13, a key cytokine in many atopic disorders, is highly correlated with many crucial genes in EoE. As seen in PheWas studies, IL-13 polymorphisms are common in EoE.[21,80,81] IL-13 has multiple cell-specific effects: it induces epithelial eotaxin-3 production, blocks DSG1 and FLG expression, and stimulates fibroblasts to express periostin.[82] In human trials, anti-IL-13 reduces tissue eosinophilia, although primary endpoints were not met.[83,84]

### Interleukin-4

IL-4 is a prototypical cytokine involved in Th2 responses. IL-4 is less abundant in EoE esophageal tissue than IL-13. These related cytokines share some receptors, but also activate receptors specific to their IL type. Only IL-4 has receptors on T helper cells[85]; IL-4, but not IL-13, can help induce Th2 cell differentiation.

### Interleukin-5

IL-5 is central to the EoE pathway because it causes eosinophil proliferation, survival, activation, and chemotaxis. IL-5 and its receptor are expressed in esophageal tissue in EoE. In animal models, eosinophils and fibrosis are decreased in the absence of IL-5. Clinical anti-IL-5 trials showed reduced esophageal eosinophil and mast cell contents, but clinical endpoints were not consistently met.[78,86–88]

### Eotaxin-3

Eotaxin-3 (CCL26) is the most abundant EoE chemokine, regardless of the patient's age, gender, and atopic status.[54,89] A single-nucleotide polymorphism in the eotaxin-3 gene is associated with EoE.[54,90,91] Topical steroids and PPIs decrease eotaxin-3 expression.[5,92]

### IgE and IgG4

Skin prick food testing and serum food-specific IgE poorly predict EoE trigger foods.[93,94] Mice devoid of B cells can still develop EoE.[64] Adequate blockade of IgE does not eradicate EoE.[95] Together, these data are strong evidence that EoE, unlike many atopic diseases, is not IgE mediated. Esophageal tissue from patients with EoE have a markedly increased IgG4 content, abundant IgG4 plasma cells in the subjacent lamina propria, and serum IgG4 antibodies to common EoE trigger foods.[95] Food-specific IgG4 is in the tissues of patients with EoE.[96] The specific contribution of IgG4 to disease has yet to be elucidated. Food-specific IgG4 presumably acts as a blocking antibody, explaining the lack of an IgE-mediated effect, but otherwise has an unclear role in EoE.

### Thymic Stromal Lymphopoeitin

TSLP and its receptor TSLPR are implicated in EoE by GWAS studies and a mouse model.[79,97] TSLP induces a type 2 immune response, particularly in the presence of basophils, probably by multiple mechanisms.

### Fibrosis and Remodeling

Over time, patients risk gradual esophageal fibrosis and strictures if EoE is not controlled.[98] IL-13, IL-4, IL-5, eotaxin-3, periostin, and TGFB1 all are suspected of contributing to this tissue remodeling.[98–100] IL-13 and TGFB1 activate quiescent fibroblasts to transdifferentiate into myofibroblasts that organize and synthesize extracellular matrix. Stromal periostin expression of EoE, triggered by IL-13 and TGFB1 in different cell lines (fibroblasts and epithelium),[101] enhances eosinophil recruitment and adhesion.[102] Both genetic and translational discoveries implicate a strong role for TGFB1 in EoE pathogenesis. TGFB1 has many effects; among them it is strongly profibrogenic, inducing myofibroblast differentiation and expression of many fibroblast activation genes and synthesis of the extracellular matrix.[103] Via SMADs, TGFB1 modulates the deposition of collagen and fibrosis. SMAD3 knockout mice are protected against EoE-related fibrosis. Remodeling is seen in pediatric and adult EoE, with smooth muscle hypertrophy and collagen deposition.[104] Matrix metalloproteinase upregulation (responsible in part for extracellular matrix degradation) is reversible with steroid therapy.[105]

## SUMMARY

EoE is an inflammatory, immune-driven disease of the esophagus that is defined by a complex relationship between immune dysfunction, genetics, and environment. Symptoms vary according to age of patient and duration of disease. Multiple cytokines and cells are likely contributory to the disease including lymphocytes, eosinophils, mast cells, basophils, eotaxin-3, IL-13, IL-5, and more. The exact cause and causative signaling in the disease onset remains elusive but likely involves a large interplay between epithelial dysfunction and antigen presentation with lymphocyte and eosinophil recruitment. For now, topical steroids and food elimination diets are a logical approach to management of disease and prevention of complications through its abilities to reduce or reverse key mechanistic abnormalities in EoE.

## REFERENCES

1. Liacouras CA, Furuta GT, Hirano I, et al. Eosinophilic esophagitis: updated consensus recommendations for children and adults. J Allergy Clin Immunol 2011;128(1):3–20.
2. Molina-Infante J, Bredenoord AJ, Cheng E, et al. Proton pump inhibitor-responsive oesophageal eosinophilia: an entity challenging current diagnostic criteria for eosinophilic oesophagitis. Gut 2016;65(3):524–31.
3. Shoda T, Matsuda A, Nomura I, et al. Eosinophilic esophagitis versus proton pump inhibitor-responsive esophageal eosinophilia: transcriptome analysis. J Allergy Clin Immunol 2017;139(6):2010–3.e4.
4. Wen T, Dellon ES, Moawad FJ, et al. Transcriptome analysis of proton pump inhibitor-responsive esophageal eosinophilia reveals proton pump inhibitor-reversible allergic inflammation. J Allergy Clin Immunol 2015;135(1):187–97.
5. Cheng E, Zhang X, Huo X, et al. Omeprazole blocks eotaxin-3 expression by oesophageal squamous cells from patients with eosinophilic oesophagitis and GORD. Gut 2013;62(6):824–32.
6. Zhang X, Cheng E, Huo X, et al. Omeprazole blocks STAT6 binding to the eotaxin-3 promoter in eosinophilic esophagitis cells. PLoS One 2012;7(11):e50037.
7. Sodikoff J, Hirano I. Proton pump inhibitor-responsive esophageal eosinophilia does not preclude food-responsive eosinophilic esophagitis. J Allergy Clin Immunol 2016;137(2):631–3.
8. DeBrosse CW, Collins MH, Buckmeier Butz BK, et al. Identification, epidemiology, and chronicity of pediatric esophageal eosinophilia, 1982-1999. J Allergy Clin Immunol 2010;126(1):112–9.
9. Collins MH, Martin LJ, Alexander ES, et al. Newly developed and validated eosinophilic esophagitis histology scoring system and evidence that it outperforms peak eosinophil count for disease diagnosis and monitoring. Dis Esophagus 2017;30(3):1–8.
10. Salek J, Clayton F, Vinson L, et al. Endoscopic appearance and location dictate diagnostic yield of biopsies in eosinophilic oesophagitis. Aliment Pharmacol Ther 2015;41(12):1288–95.
11. Protheroe C, Woodruff SA, de Petris G, et al. A novel histologic scoring system to evaluate mucosal biopsies from patients with eosinophilic esophagitis. Clin Gastroenterol Hepatol 2009;7(7):749–55.e11.
12. D'Alessandro A, Esposito D, Pesce M, et al. Eosinophilic esophagitis: from pathophysiology to treatment. World J Gastrointest Pathophysiol 2015;6(4):150–8.

13. Safroneeva E, Coslovsky M, Kuehni CE, et al. Eosinophilic oesophagitis: relationship of quality of life with clinical, endoscopic and histological activity. Aliment Pharmacol Ther 2015;42(8):1000–10.
14. van Rhijn BD, Smout AJ, Bredenoord AJ. Disease duration determines health-related quality of life in adult eosinophilic esophagitis patients. Neurogastroenterol Motil 2014;26(6):772–8.
15. Byrne KR, Panagiotakis PH, Hilden K, et al. Retrospective analysis of esophageal food impaction: differences in etiology by age and gender. Dig Dis Sci 2007;52(3):717–21.
16. Lynch KL, Dhalla S, Chedid V, et al. Gender is a determinative factor in the initial clinical presentation of eosinophilic esophagitis. Dis Esophagus 2016;174–8.
17. Larsson H, Norder Grusell E, Tegtmeyer B, et al. Grade of eosinophilia versus symptoms in patients with dysphagia and esophageal eosinophilia. Dis Esophagus 2016;29(8):971–6.
18. Safroneeva E, Straumann A, Coslovsky M, et al. Symptoms have modest accuracy in detecting endoscopic and histologic remission in adults with eosinophilic esophagitis. Gastroenterology 2016;150(3):581–90.e4.
19. Sleiman PM, March M, Hakonarson H. The genetic basis of eosinophilic esophagitis. Best Pract Res Clin Gastroenterol 2015;29(5):701–7.
20. Sleiman PM, Wang ML, Cianferoni A, et al. GWAS identifies four novel eosinophilic esophagitis loci. Nat Commun 2014;5:5593.
21. Namjou B, Marsolo K, Caroll RJ, et al. Phenome-wide association study (PheWAS) in EMR-linked pediatric cohorts, genetically links PLCL1 to speech language development and IL5-IL13 to eosinophilic esophagitis. Front Genet 2014;5:401.
22. D'Mello RJ, Caldwell JM, Azouz NP, et al. LRRC31 is induced by IL-13 and regulates kallikrein expression and barrier function in the esophageal epithelium. Mucosal Immunol 2016;9(3):744–56.
23. Amaral AF, Minelli C, Guerra S, et al. The locus C11orf30 increases susceptibility to poly-sensitization. Allergy 2015;70(3):328–33.
24. Krishnamurthy P, Kaplan MH. STAT6 and PARP family members in the development of T Cell-dependent allergic inflammation. Immune Netw 2016;16(4):201–10.
25. Cheng E, Zhang X, Wilson KS, et al. JAK-STAT6 pathway inhibitors block eotaxin-3 secretion by epithelial cells and fibroblasts from esophageal eosinophilia patients: promising agents to improve inflammation and prevent fibrosis in EoE. PLoS One 2016;11(6):e0157376.
26. Kottyan LC, Davis BP, Sherrill JD, et al. Genome-wide association analysis of eosinophilic esophagitis provides insight into the tissue specificity of this allergic disease. Nat Genet 2014;46(8):895–900.
27. Davis BP, Stucke EM, Khorki ME, et al. Eosinophilic esophagitis-linked calpain 14 is an IL-13-induced protease that mediates esophageal epithelial barrier impairment. JCI Insight 2016;1(4):e86355.
28. Litosh VA, Rochman M, Rymer JK, et al. Calpain-14 and its association with eosinophilic esophagitis. J Allergy Clin Immunol 2017;139(6):1762–71.e7.
29. Sherrill JD, Kc K, Wu D, et al. Desmoglein-1 regulates esophageal epithelial barrier function and immune responses in eosinophilic esophagitis. Mucosal Immunol 2014;7(3):718–29.
30. Kottyan LC, Rothenberg ME. Genetics of eosinophilic esophagitis. Mucosal Immunol 2017;10(3):580–8.

31. Allen-Brady K, Firszt R, Fang JC, et al. Population-based familial aggregation of eosinophilic esophagitis suggests a genetic contribution. J Allergy Clin Immunol 2017. [Epub ahead of print].

32. Olson AA, Evans MD, Johansson MW, et al. Role of food and aeroallergen sensitization in eosinophilic esophagitis in adults. Ann Allergy Asthma Immunol 2016; 117(4):387–93.e2.

33. Slae M, Persad R, Leung AJ, et al. Role of environmental factors in the development of pediatric eosinophilic esophagitis. Dig Dis Sci 2015;60(11):3364–72.

34. Green DJ, Cotton CC, Dellon ES. The role of environmental exposures in the etiology of eosinophilic esophagitis: a systematic review. Mayo Clin Proc 2015; 90(10):1400–10.

35. Benninger MS, Strohl M, Holy CE, et al. Prevalence of atopic disease in patients with eosinophilic esophagitis. Int Forum Allergy Rhinol 2017;7(8):757–62.

36. Peterson KA, Byrne KR, Vinson LA, et al. Elemental diet induces histologic response in adult eosinophilic esophagitis. Am J Gastroenterol 2013;108(5): 759–66.

37. Warners MJ, Vlieg-Boerstra BJ, Verheij J, et al. Esophageal and small intestinal mucosal integrity in eosinophilic esophagitis and response to an elemental diet. Am J Gastroenterol 2017;112(7):1061–71.

38. Cotton CC, Eluri S, Wolf WA, et al. Six-food elimination diet and topical steroids are effective for eosinophilic esophagitis: a meta-regression. Dig Dis Sci 2017. [Epub ahead of print].

39. Kagalwalla AF, Wechsler JB, Amsden K, et al. Efficacy of a 4-food elimination diet for children with eosinophilic esophagitis. Clin Gastroenterol Hepatol 2017. [Epub ahead of print].

40. Jensen ET, Bertelsen RJ. Assessing early life factors for eosinophilic esophagitis: lessons from other allergic diseases. Curr Treat Options Gastroenterol 2016; 14(1):39–50.

41. Jensen ET, Dellon ES. Environmental and infectious factors in eosinophilic esophagitis. Best Pract Res Clin Gastroenterol 2015;29(5):721–9.

42. Radano MC, Yuan Q, Katz A, et al. Cesarean section and antibiotic use found to be associated with eosinophilic esophagitis. J Allergy Clin Immunol Pract 2014; 2(4):475–7.e1.

43. Mansoor E, Cooper GS. The 2010-2015 prevalence of eosinophilic esophagitis in the USA: a population-based study. Dig Dis Sci 2016;61(10):2928–34.

44. Jensen ET, Hoffman K, Shaheen NJ, et al. Esophageal eosinophilia is increased in rural areas with low population density: results from a national pathology database. Am J Gastroenterol 2014;109(5):668–75.

45. von Arnim U, Wex T, Link A, et al. *Helicobacter pylori* infection is associated with a reduced risk of developing eosinophilic oesophagitis. Aliment Pharmacol Ther 2016;43(7):825–30.

46. Dellon ES, Peery AF, Shaheen NJ, et al. Inverse association of esophageal eosinophilia with *Helicobacter pylori* based on analysis of a US pathology database. Gastroenterology 2011;141(5):1586–92.

47. Lucendo AJ, Molina-Infante J, Arias A, et al. Seasonal variation in the diagnosis of eosinophilic esophagitis: there and back again. J Pediatr Gastroenterol Nutr 2017;64(1):e25.

48. Warners MJ, van Rhijn BD, Verheij J, et al. Disease activity in eosinophilic esophagitis is associated with impaired esophageal barrier integrity. Am J Physiol Gastrointest Liver Physiol 2017;313(3):G230–8.

49. Patel DA, Vaezi MF. Utility of esophageal mucosal impedance as a diagnostic test for esophageal disease. Curr Opin Gastroenterol 2017;33(4):277–84.
50. Katzka DA, Ravi K, Geno DM, et al. Endoscopic mucosal impedance measurements correlate with eosinophilia and dilation of intercellular spaces in patients with eosinophilic esophagitis. Clin Gastroenterol Hepatol 2015;13(7):1242–8.e1.
51. van Rhijn BD, Kessing BF, Smout AJ, et al. Oesophageal baseline impedance values are decreased in patients with eosinophilic oesophagitis. United European Gastroenterol J 2013;1(4):242–8.
52. Pothoven KL, Norton JE, Hulse KE, et al. Oncostatin M promotes mucosal epithelial barrier dysfunction, and its expression is increased in patients with eosinophilic mucosal disease. J Allergy Clin Immunol 2015;136(3):737–46.e4.
53. Politi E, Angelakopoulou A, Grapsa D, et al. Filaggrin and periostin expression is altered in eosinophilic esophagitis and normalized with treatment. J Pediatr Gastroenterol Nutr 2017;65(1):47–52.
54. Blanchard C, Wang N, Stringer KF, et al. Eotaxin-3 and a uniquely conserved gene-expression profile in eosinophilic esophagitis. J Clin Invest 2006;116(2):536–47.
55. Le-Carlson M, Seki S, Abarbanel D, et al. Markers of antigen presentation and activation on eosinophils and T cells in the esophageal tissue of patients with eosinophilic esophagitis. J Pediatr Gastroenterol Nutr 2013;56(3):257–62.
56. Lingblom C, Bergquist H, Johnsson M, et al. Topical corticosteroids do not revert the activated phenotype of eosinophils in eosinophilic esophagitis but decrease surface levels of CD18 resulting in diminished adherence to ICAM-1, ICAM-2, and endothelial cells. Inflammation 2014;37(6):1932–44.
57. Nguyen T, Gernez Y, Fuentebella J, et al. Immunophenotyping of peripheral eosinophils demonstrates activation in eosinophilic esophagitis. J Pediatr Gastroenterol Nutr 2011;53(1):40–7.
58. Saffari H, Hoffman LH, Peterson KA, et al. Electron microscopy elucidates eosinophil degranulation patterns in patients with eosinophilic esophagitis. J Allergy Clin Immunol 2014;133(6):1728–34.e1.
59. Peterson KA, Cobell WJ, Clayton FC, et al. Extracellular eosinophil granule protein deposition in ringed esophagus with sparse eosinophils. Dig Dis Sci 2015;60(9):2646–53.
60. Kephart GM, Alexander JA, Arora AS, et al. Marked deposition of eosinophil-derived neurotoxin in adult patients with eosinophilic esophagitis. Am J Gastroenterol 2010;105(2):298–307.
61. Patel AJ, Fuentebella J, Gernez Y, et al. Increased HLA-DR expression on tissue eosinophils in eosinophilic esophagitis. J Pediatr Gastroenterol Nutr 2010;51(3):290–4.
62. Mulder DJ, Pacheco I, Hurlbut DJ, et al. FGF9-induced proliferative response to eosinophilic inflammation in oesophagitis. Gut 2009;58(2):166–73.
63. Lucendo AJ, Navarro M, Comas C, et al. Immunophenotypic characterization and quantification of the epithelial inflammatory infiltrate in eosinophilic esophagitis through stereology: an analysis of the cellular mechanisms of the disease and the immunologic capacity of the esophagus. Am J Surg Pathol 2007;31(4):598–606.
64. Mishra A, Schlotman J, Wang M, et al. Critical role for adaptive T cell immunity in experimental eosinophilic esophagitis in mice. J Leukoc Biol 2007;81(4):916–24.
65. Mitson-Salazar A, Yin Y, Wansley DL, et al. Hematopoietic prostaglandin D synthase defines a proeosinophilic pathogenic effector human T(H)2 cell subpopulation with enhanced function. J Allergy Clin Immunol 2016;137(3):907–18.e9.

66. Tantibhaedhyangkul U, Tatevian N, Gilger MA, et al. Increased esophageal regulatory T cells and eosinophil characteristics in children with eosinophilic esophagitis and gastroesophageal reflux disease. Ann Clin Lab Sci 2009;39(2): 99–107.

67. Stuck MC, Straumann A, Simon HU. Relative lack of T regulatory cells in adult eosinophilic esophagitis: no normalization after corticosteroid therapy. Allergy 2011;66(5):705–7.

68. Jyonouchi S, Smith CL, Saretta F, et al. Invariant natural killer T cells in children with eosinophilic esophagitis. Clin Exp Allergy 2014;44(1):58–68.

69. Rayapudi M, Rajavelu P, Zhu X, et al. Invariant natural killer T-cell neutralization is a possible novel therapy for human eosinophilic esophagitis. Clin Transl Immunology 2014;3(1):e9.

70. Lexmond WS, Neves JF, Nurko S, et al. Involvement of the iNKT cell pathway is associated with early-onset eosinophilic esophagitis and response to allergen avoidance therapy. Am J Gastroenterol 2014;109(5):646–57.

71. Doherty TA, Baum R, Newbury RO, et al. Group 2 innate lymphocytes (ILC2) are enriched in active eosinophilic esophagitis. J Allergy Clin Immunol 2015;136(3): 792–4.e3.

72. Niranjan R, Mavi P, Rayapudi M, et al. Pathogenic role of mast cells in experimental eosinophilic esophagitis. Am J Physiol Gastrointest Liver Physiol 2013; 304(12):G1087–94.

73. Mulder DJ, Mak N, Hurlbut DJ, et al. Atopic and non-atopic eosinophilic oesophagitis are distinguished by immunoglobulin E-bearing intraepithelial mast cells. Histopathology 2012;61(5):810–22.

74. Aceves SS, Chen D, Newbury RO, et al. Mast cells infiltrate the esophageal smooth muscle in patients with eosinophilic esophagitis, express TGF-beta1, and increase esophageal smooth muscle contraction. J Allergy Clin Immunol 2010;126(6):1198–204.e4.

75. Abonia JP, Blanchard C, Butz BB, et al. Involvement of mast cells in eosinophilic esophagitis. J Allergy Clin Immunol 2010;126(1):140–9.

76. Abonia JP, Franciosi JP, Rothenberg ME. TGF-beta1: mediator of a feedback loop in eosinophilic esophagitis–or should we really say mastocytic esophagitis? J Allergy Clin Immunol 2010;126(6):1205–7.

77. Wang YH, Hogan SP, Fulkerson PC, et al. Expanding the paradigm of eosinophilic esophagitis: mast cells and IL-9. J Allergy Clin Immunol 2013;131(6): 1583–5.

78. Otani IM, Anilkumar AA, Newbury RO, et al. Anti-IL-5 therapy reduces mast cell and IL-9 cell numbers in pediatric patients with eosinophilic esophagitis. J Allergy Clin Immunol 2013;131(6):1576–82.

79. Noti M, Wojno ED, Kim BS, et al. Thymic stromal lymphopoietin-elicited basophil responses promote eosinophilic esophagitis. Nat Med 2013;19(8):1005–13.

80. Blanchard C, Stucke EM, Burwinkel K, et al. Coordinate interaction between IL-13 and epithelial differentiation cluster genes in eosinophilic esophagitis. J Immunol 2010;184(7):4033–41.

81. Blanchard C, Mingler MK, Vicario M, et al. IL-13 involvement in eosinophilic esophagitis: transcriptome analysis and reversibility with glucocorticoids. J Allergy Clin Immunol 2007;120(6):1292–300.

82. Zuo L, Fulkerson PC, Finkelman FD, et al. IL-13 induces esophageal remodeling and gene expression by an eosinophil-independent, IL-13R alpha 2-inhibited pathway. J Immunol 2010;185(1):660–9.

83. Niranjan R, Rayapudi M, Mishra A, et al. Pathogenesis of allergen-induced eosinophilic esophagitis is independent of interleukin (IL)-13. Immunol Cell Biol 2013;91(6):408–15.
84. Rothenberg ME, Wen T, Greenberg A, et al. Intravenous anti-IL-13 mAb QAX576 for the treatment of eosinophilic esophagitis. J Allergy Clin Immunol 2015; 135(2):500–7.
85. Zurawski G, de Vries JE. Interleukin 13, an interleukin 4-like cytokine that acts on monocytes and B cells, but not on T cells. Immunol Today 1994;15(1):19–26.
86. Spergel JM, Rothenberg ME, Collins MH, et al. Reslizumab in children and adolescents with eosinophilic esophagitis: results of a double-blind, randomized, placebo-controlled trial. J Allergy Clin Immunol 2012;129(2):456–63, 463.e1–3.
87. Assa'ad AH, Gupta SK, Collins MH, et al. An antibody against IL-5 reduces numbers of esophageal intraepithelial eosinophils in children with eosinophilic esophagitis. Gastroenterology 2011;141(5):1593–604.
88. Straumann A, Conus S, Grzonka P, et al. Anti-interleukin-5 antibody treatment (mepolizumab) in active eosinophilic oesophagitis: a randomised, placebo-controlled, double-blind trial. Gut 2010;59(1):21–30.
89. Sherrill JD, Kiran KC, Blanchard C, et al. Analysis and expansion of the eosinophilic esophagitis transcriptome by RNA sequencing. Genes Immun 2014;15(6): 361–9.
90. Moawad FJ, Wells JM, Johnson RL, et al. Comparison of eotaxin-3 biomarker in patients with eosinophilic oesophagitis, proton pump inhibitor-responsive oesophageal eosinophilia and gastro-oesophageal reflux disease. Aliment Pharmacol Ther 2015;42(2):231–8.
91. Romano C, Chiaro A, Lucarelli S, et al. Mucosal cytokine profiles in paediatric eosinophilic oesophagitis: a case-control study. Dig Liver Dis 2014;46(7):590–5.
92. Lucendo AJ, De Rezende L, Comas C, et al. Treatment with topical steroids downregulates IL-5, eotaxin-1/CCL11, and eotaxin-3/CCL26 gene expression in eosinophilic esophagitis. Am J Gastroenterol 2008;103(9):2184–93.
93. Hill DA, Dudley JW, Spergel JM. The prevalence of eosinophilic esophagitis in pediatric patients with IgE-mediated food allergy. J Allergy Clin Immunol Pract 2017;5(2):369–75.
94. Aceves SS. Allergy testing in patients with eosinophilic esophagitis. Gastroenterol Hepatol 2016;12(8):516–8.
95. Clayton F, Fang JC, Gleich GJ, et al. Eosinophilic esophagitis in adults is associated with IgG4 and not mediated by IgE. Gastroenterology 2014;147(3): 602–9.
96. Wright BL, Kulis M, Gu R, et al. Food-specific IgG4 is associated with eosinophilic esophagitis. J Allergy Clin Immunol 2016;138(4):1190–2.e3.
97. Sherrill JD, Gao PS, Stucke EM, et al. Variants of thymic stromal lymphopoietin and its receptor associate with eosinophilic esophagitis. J Allergy Clin Immunol 2010;126(1):160–5.e3.
98. Schoepfer AM, Safroneeva E, Bussmann C, et al. Delay in diagnosis of eosinophilic esophagitis increases risk for stricture formation in a time-dependent manner. Gastroenterology 2013;145(6):1230–6.e1-2.
99. Dellon ES, Kim HP, Sperry SL, et al. A phenotypic analysis shows that eosinophilic esophagitis is a progressive fibrostenotic disease. Gastrointest Endosc 2014;79(4):577–85.e4.
100. Li-Kim-Moy JP, Tobias V, Day AS, et al. Esophageal subepithelial fibrosis and hyalinization are features of eosinophilic esophagitis. J Pediatr Gastroenterol Nutr 2011;52(2):147–53.

101. Nguyen N, Furuta GT, Masterson JC. Deeper than the epithelium: role of matrix and fibroblasts in pediatric and adult eosinophilic esophagitis. J Pediatr Gastroenterol Nutr 2016;63(2):168–9.
102. Blanchard C, Mingler MK, McBride M, et al. Periostin facilitates eosinophil tissue infiltration in allergic lung and esophageal responses. Mucosal Immunol 2008; 1(4):289–96.
103. Rawson R, Yang T, Newbury RO, et al. TGF-beta1-induced PAI-1 contributes to a profibrotic network in patients with eosinophilic esophagitis. J Allergy Clin Immunol 2016;138(3):791–800.e4.
104. Cho JY, Doshi A, Rosenthal P, et al. Smad3-deficient mice have reduced esophageal fibrosis and angiogenesis in a model of egg-induced eosinophilic esophagitis. J Pediatr Gastroenterol Nutr 2014;59(1):10–6.
105. Beppu L, Yang T, Luk M, et al. MMPs-2 and -14 are elevated in eosinophilic esophagitis and reduced following topical corticosteroid therapy. J Pediatr Gastroenterol Nutr 2015;61(2):194–9.

# Eosinophilic Esophagitis
## Incidence and Prevalence

Fouad J. Moawad, MD

## KEYWORDS

- Eosinophilic esophagitis • Epidemiology • Prevalence • Incidence

## KEY POINTS

- Eosinophilic esophagitis (EoE) is an emerging allergy-mediated condition that affects all ages. The clinical presentation of EoE differs between children and adults.
- The epidemiology of EoE has been reported in studies from multiple countries with varying estimates, depending on factors, such as method of data collection and populations studied.
- The incidence of EoE has increased over the years. The current estimated annual incidence is approximately 10/100,000 cases.
- The overall prevalence of EoE ranges from 10 to 57 cases/100,000 persons and is higher among symptomatic patients.

## INTRODUCTION

Eosinophilic esophagitis (EoE) is a relatively new condition first described less than 4 decades ago.[1] Since its initial description, there has been an immense interest in EoE in both the research and the clinical setting. EoE is an allergic-mediated condition that triggers an inflammatory response that leads to esophageal dysfunction, namely dysphagia and food impaction in adults, and is characterized by dense eosinophilic infiltration of the esophageal mucosa.[2,3] Several studies from multiple countries have described the epidemiology of EoE in children and adults during the past 2 decades.[4] Some of these studies are population based from geographic confined regions, whereas others are institution based using registry data and electronic medical records.

Incidence and prevalence are important aspects in understanding the epidemiology of a disease, particularly a new disease. They are both considered measures of frequency. The incidence of a condition is defined as the number of new cases in which patients who were initially free of a condition developed the condition during a set

Disclosure Statement: The author has no disclosures.
Division of Gastroenterology, Scripps Clinic, Anderson Medical Pavilion, 9898 Genesee Avenue, La Jolla, CA 92037, USA
E-mail address: Moawad.Fouad@Scrippshealth.org

Gastrointest Endoscopy Clin N Am 28 (2018) 15–25
http://dx.doi.org/10.1016/j.giec.2017.07.001
1052-5157/18/© 2017 Elsevier Inc. All rights reserved.

period of time. The prevalence is defined as the total proportion of patients with a condition over time. Therefore, in chronic conditions, such as EoE, the prevalence is typically greater than the incidence because it includes new cases as well as those known over time. Both are typically reported as a fraction of a population at risk (eg, per 100,000 individuals). One important difference between incidence and prevalence is that in incidence, an interval period is followed over time to determine new cases that have developed, whereas prevalence is described at a given point in time. Incidence describes the rate of acquiring a condition, and prevalence refers to how widespread a condition is.

## INCIDENCE OF EOSINOPHILIC ESOPHAGITIS

One important question regarding the incidence of EoE is whether an increase in the number of new cases truly exists or if the observed increase in incidence is from a higher awareness of the condition, improved recognition by gastroenterologists, and therefore, more esophageal biopsies being taken. The answer is likely a combination of both, increased awareness and a true increase in number of new cases. In one study, the increasing incidence appeared to be explained by a higher number of esophageal biopsies taken over a 4-year period.[5] More recent studies, however, suggest an actual increase in the number of cases that cannot simply be explained by an increase in esophageal biopsies.[6,7] Overall, the incidence of EoE ranges from 0.7/100,000 to 10.7/100,000 depending on the population studied and the method of data collection, that is, by using institutional electronic medical records and databases, International Classification of Diseases (ICD) codes (530.13), or nationwide registries.

In a population-based study in Denmark using a national pathology registry over a 15-year period, the incidence of EoE increased from 0.13/100,000 to 2.6/100,000, representing a nearly 20-fold increase. One important aspect of this study was determining that esophageal biopsies increased only 2-fold over the same time period, suggesting that an increase in awareness and recognition alone could not account for the increase in incidence noted.[6] The incidence reported in this study was higher than a previous study from Denmark where the incidence was 1.6/100,000.[8] There are some notable differences between these 2 studies. The study with the lower incidence rate was limited to children and from the southern region of the country over a 3-year period, whereas the more recent study was all inclusive of the entire Danish population.[8]

There have been several additional European population-based studies that have reported the incidence of EoE. In a defined region in Switzerland with a population of 90,000 cared for by 2 gastroenterologists and one pathologist, the incidence of EoE was 2.45/100,000.[7] The incidence remained stable from 1989 to 2001, but an increase was observed from 2004 to 2009. Although there certainly was an increase in upper endoscopies performed over the years, the number of new EoE cases was higher than the number of endoscopies during that same time period, suggesting an increase in the actual incidence of EoE. In another study from the Western part of Switzerland, in which there are nearly 750,000 inhabitants, the incidence of EoE was calculated based on review of pathology databases to identify any cases of esophageal eosinophilia followed by chart review to ensure an accurate diagnosis of EoE. The incidence increased from 0.16/100,000 cases in 2004 to 6.3/100,000 in 2013.[9] In another population-based study from the Netherlands in which pathology reports from a nationwide registry were used to identify cases of esophageal eosinophilia over a 15-year period, the incidence of EoE increased from 0.01/100,000 to 1.31/100,000.[10] The highest incidence observed was between the ages of 20 and 29 years. One limitation of this study was that the definition of EoE was strictly pathologic and there were no data on the exact number of eosinophils, therefore possibly overestimating the true incidence of EoE. In a retrospective study that included 2 hospitals in Spain, the incidence of EoE in individuals aged 16 and older was 6.37/100,000 over a 6-year period.[11] In Slovenia, the incidence of EoE in pediatric patients was noted to increase 6-fold over an 8-year period from 0.2/100,000 to 1.8/100,000.[12]

The increase in incidence has also been observed in a population-based study from Canada.[5] Using an endoscopy and pathology database, the incidence increased from 2.1/100,000 to 11/100,000, representing a greater than 5-fold increase in incidence rate. Similar trends have been reported in Hamilton, Ohio, where the incidence in children increased from 9.1/100,000 to 12.8/100,000 from 2000 to 2003 with an average incidence of 10.7/100,000.[13] In a fixed population of approximately 120,000 persons in Olmstead County, Minnesota, where most hospital and outpatient visits are captured in a registry, the incidence of EoE increased from 0.35/100,000 between 1991 and 1995 to 9.4/100,000 1 decade later. All cases of suspected EoE were reviewed by a gastrointestinal pathologist, and EoE was defined by the presence of $\geq$15 eosinophils per high-power field. Although there was an increase in new EoE diagnoses over time, the investigators also noted a parallel increase in the number of endoscopies during the same time period[14] (**Fig. 1**).

In a US military population that was enrolled in a single electronic medical record system that included nearly 7.8 million active duty members, their dependents, and retirees, cases of EoE were identified using ICD-9 codes. Veteran Affairs (VA) patients were excluded from this cohort. The incidence of EoE was found to be 4.8/100,000.[15] In another population study from the United States, health insurance claims were explored over a 3-year period. The incidence of EoE in 11.5 million individuals was 18.8/100,000.[16]

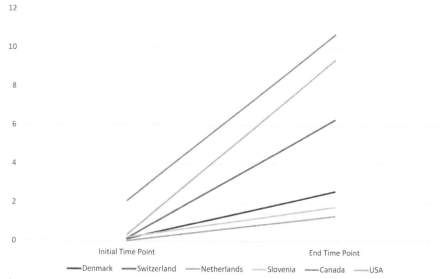

**Fig. 1.** An increase in incidence of EoE per 100,000 individuals is observed in several studies from North America and Europe.

One institution in West Virginia reported the incidence of EoE in children as 0.73/ 100,000, which is much lower than other population-based studies that had larger and more diverse populations. In this study, endoscopy records were reviewed over a 10-year period, and 25% of cases were randomly selected from each year for review of histology. The incidence was likely underestimated because the referral area for the practice was limited to a small region.[17] In a New Zealand study aimed to assess the incidence among a cohort of patients presenting with dysphagia, the incidence was reported at 14.1% of patients having esophageal biopsies.[18]

## PREVALENCE OF EOSINOPHILIC ESOPHAGITIS

Some studies have described the prevalence of EoE among patients undergoing upper endoscopy for symptoms, whereas other studies reported the prevalence of EoE in a general population. Many population-based studies have estimated the prevalence of EoE using data from either electronic medical records, ICD codes, or nationwide registries. The prevalence rates in these studies range from 10/100,000 to 57/100,000.

### Eosinophilic Esophagitis Among Symptomatic Patients

The prevalence of EoE is higher among patients who have nonesophageal symptoms compared with the general population and continues to increase in patients with esophageal symptoms, particularly those with dysphagia and food impaction, especially because EoE has become one of the most common causes of these presentations.[19–22]

In a US military population with 400 consecutive patients presenting for upper endoscopy for various reasons, the prevalence of EoE, defined as ≥20 eosinophils per high-power field, was 6.5%.[23] However, this study likely overestimated the true prevalence in this population, because not all patients had esophageal symptoms, which is an essential part of the diagnosis.[2] These results were very similar to a Korean study in which the prevalence was 6.6% in patients presenting with various upper gastrointestinal complaints.[24] The prevalence was lower in a VA study in patients presenting for an elective endoscopy in which at least 1 esophageal biopsy was taken. In these patients, the prevalence of EoE was 2.3%. However, the prevalence was reported as 0.66% when strict criteria were used for diagnosis, that is, the presence of dysphagia, greater than 15 eosinophils per high-power field in the setting of an adequate course of acid suppressants.[25] In a single-center Turkish population, the prevalence of EoE was 2.6%, with heartburn being the most common symptom.[26] EoE has been described less frequently in Hispanics than Caucasians.[27] In a population from Southeastern Mexico undergoing upper endoscopy, the prevalence was reported in 1.7%. In this study, EoE patients were more likely to present with dysphagia and have asthma.[28]

In a Chinese population undergoing endoscopy for various indications where biopsies were reviewed, the prevalence of EoE was 0.34%.[29] Most diagnosed patients presented with dysphagia, and the prevalence among men and women was similar. In a Japanese study of more than 23,000 patients who had endoscopy for symptoms or as part of an annual checkup, the prevalence was 17.1/100,000 (0.17%).[30] The question whether EoE is truly less prevalent in Asian countries due to genetic differences versus a lower frequency explained by study designs is yet to be determined, although the gene expression profiles between Japanese and US patients with EoE were similar in a small case control study.[31] In addition, the demographics, clinical presentation, and prevalence of atopic conditions among Asian patients were similar to characteristics of EoE patients from Western countries.[32]

### Eosinophilic Esophagitis in Patients With Refractory Reflux

Most studies reporting the prevalence of EoE in patients with refractory reflux symptoms are performed in adult populations with a prevalence ranging between 0.8% and 9%[33–35]; therefore, it is reasonable to take multiple esophageal biopsies when performing upper endoscopy in individuals presenting with refractory reflux symptoms even when the classic endoscopic features of EoE are not present. In one study, EoE patients were more likely to also report dysphagia and have coexisting atopic conditions.[36]

### Eosinophilic Esophagitis in Patients With Dysphagia

In patients presenting with dysphagia, EoE is a common cause with a prevalence ranging between 15% and 23%. In a study from the Mayo Clinic in which patients with dysphagia without obvious endoscopic causes had esophageal biopsies, the prevalence of EoE was 15%.[37] In a similar study where patients presenting with dysphagia had upper endoscopy with biopsies taken from the middle and distal esophagus, 12% met criteria for EoE. These patients were more likely to be younger and have coexisting atopic conditions.[38] EoE was commonly found in 2 other prospective cohort studies in patients presenting with dysphagia. In one study in which patients with nonobstructive dysphagia were prospectively enrolled and underwent esophageal biopsies, the prevalence of EoE was 22%.[39] Most patients diagnosed were Caucasian men. In another cohort of patients presenting with dysphagia, esophageal eosinophilia was present in 38%, and after a proton-pump inhibitor (PPI) trial, EoE was diagnosed in 23% of patients.[40]

### Eosinophilic Esophagitis in Patients With Food Impaction

Because EoE is the most frequent cause of food impaction, particularly in a younger population, the reported prevalence of EoE in patients presenting with this chief complaint is high and ranges from 46% to 63%.[19,41–43] Although food impaction is more likely to be reported in adults, 2 studies included children in their cohort. In one study at a tertiary care center where the patient population ranged from 1 month to 18 years of age, 76% of patients had esophageal inflammation on biopsies.[43] In another study with a mixed population of children and adults, EoE was found in 46% of patients who presented with an esophageal food or foreign body impaction. Adults were more likely to have food impactions compared with children, who had nonfood impactions (eg, toys and coins).[19] A recent study from Sweden explored the prevalence of EoE among adult patients presenting with food bolus impaction. EoE was detected in 18% of patients, whereas another 22% had both EoE and lymphocytic esophagitis[44] (**Table 1**).

### Eosinophilic Esophagitis in Population-Based Studies

In population-based studies, the prevalence of EoE varies widely. In 2 European studies, one from Southern Denmark and the other from the Netherlands, the prevalence is relatively low, reported between 2.3 and 4.1/100,000.[8,10] The study by Dalby and colleagues[8] was restricted to one region of Denmark and to a pediatric population. A recently updated epidemiology study inclusive of the general population and the entire country reported a prevalence of 13.8/100,000.[6] Which is likely a better estimate of the true prevalence of EoE in Denmark. This prevalence rate is consistent

**Table 1**
The prevalence of eosinophilic esophagitis in population-based studies ranges between approximately 10/100,000 and 57/100,000

| Author, y | Country | Population Size | Population Type | Number of EoE Cases | Time Period | Prevalence per 100,000 |
|---|---|---|---|---|---|---|
| Ally et al,[15] 2015 | US | 10,180,515 | Adults and children | 987 | 2008–2009 | 9.7 |
| Arias & Lucendo,[11] 2013 | Spain | 89,642 | Adults | 40 | 2005–2011 | 44.6 |
| Dellon,[16] 2014 | US | 35,575,388 | Adults and children | 6513 | 2009–2011 | 56.7 |
| Dellon et al,[6] 2015 | Denmark | 5,500,000 | Adults and children | 844 | 1997–2012 | 13.8 |
| Giriens et al,[9] 2015 | Switzerland | 743,317 | Adults and children | 179 | 1993–2013 | 24.1 |
| Hruz et al,[7] 2011 | Switzerland | 90,000 | Adults | 46 | 1989–2009 | 42.8 |
| Kim et al,[49] 2015 | US | 3,486,069 | Adults and children | 1561 | 2008–2013 | 45.0 |
| Mansoor & Cooper,[46] 2015 | US | 30,301,440 | Adults and children | 7840 | 1999–2015 | 25.9 |
| Maradey-Romero et al,[47] 2015 | US | 9,559,570 | Adults and children | 4840 | 2011–2014 | 50.6 |
| Prasad et al,[14] 2009 | US | 120,000 | Adults and children | 78 | 1976–2005 | 55.0 |
| Syed et al,[5] 2012 | Canada | 1,250,000 | Adults and children | 421 | 2004–2008 | 33.7 |

with 3 additional studies, 2 from pediatric populations and one from a US military population.[15,17,45]

Other studies estimate a higher prevalence of EoE ranging between 24 and 57/100,000.[6,9,46] In one US population-based study using a large database that included records from 26 health care systems and more than 30 million individuals over a 5-year period, the prevalence of EoE was estimated to be 25.9/100,000.[46] Similar to many other studies, the prevalence was higher in Caucasian men. In this study, the investigators added PPI exposure in the search criteria to eliminate PPI-responsive esophageal eosinophilia cases; however, the true prevalence may have been underestimated because subjects using over-the-counter PPI were missed by the algorithm in their search strategy. This frequency is consistent with population studies from Canada (33.7/100,000),[11] Spain (44.6/100,000),[5] Switzerland (24.1–42.8/100,000),[7] and the United States (45–56.7/100,000)[14,16,47–49] (**Tables 2 and 3**).

**Table 2**
The prevalence of eosinophilic esophagitis in population-based studies exclusively in children ranges between approximately 2/100,000 and 9/100,000

| Author, y | Country | Population Size | Number of EoE Cases | Time Period | Prevalence per 100,000 |
|---|---|---|---|---|---|
| Cherian et al,[45] 2006 | Australia | Not Reported | 285 | 1995–2004 | 8.9 |
| Gill et al,[17] 2007 | US | 60,000 | 44 | 1995–2004 | 7.3 |
| Dalby et al,[8] 2010 | Denmark | 256,164 | 6 | 2005–2007 | 2.3 |

**Table 3**
Among patients with dysphagia, the prevalence of eosinophilic esophagitis ranges between 12% and 23%, whereas among those with food impaction, the prevalence is between 40% and 55%

| Author, y | Presenting Symptom | Population Type | Number of EoE Cases | Prevalence per 100 |
|---|---|---|---|---|
| Prasad et al,[37] 2007 | Dysphagia | Adults | 33 | 15 |
| MacKenzie et al,[38] 2008 | Dysphagia | Adults | 31 | 12 |
| Ricker et al,[39] 2011 | Dysphagia | Adults | 22 | 22 |
| Dellon,[40] 2013 | Dysphagia | Adults | 40 | 23 |
| Kerlin et al,[42] 2007 | Food impaction | Adults | 14 | 50 |
| Desai et al,[41] 2005 | Food impaction | Adults | 17 | 55 |
| Hurtado et al,[43] 2011 | Food impaction | Children | 5 | 41 |
| Sperry et al,[19] 2011 | Food impaction | Adults and children | 51 | 46 |
| Truskaite & Dlugosz,[44] 2016 | Food impaction | Adults | 75 | 40 |

In a study from Northern Sweden in which endoscopy was performed on 1000 random individuals with biopsies taken from 2 locations, the squamocolumnar junction (SCJ) and 2 cm above the SCJ.[50] There were 4 patients (0.4%) who had greater than 20 eosinophils per high-power field; however, in only 1 patient was this degree of eosinophils seen when biopsies where taken above the SCJ. Furthermore, 3 of the 4 patients reported reflux symptom and not dysphagia. Therefore, given the small sample size and the lack of adhering to diagnostic criteria, the prevalence of EoE (0.4%) reported in the studyx was overestimated.

### Eosinophilic Esophagitis Associated With Other Conditions and Changes in Environments

EoE has been reported in higher prevalence in patients with connective tissue disorders[51] and autoimmune conditions, such as systemic sclerosis and celiac disease,[52–54] and recently has been associated with hypertrophic cardiomyopathy.[55] These associations may be explained by genetic susceptibilities. EoE has also been reported in higher prevalence in cold and arid environments.[56] Some studies have reported a seasonal distribution of diagnoses, possibly because of higher exposure to aeroallergens.[57,58]

### SUMMARY

EoE is an increasingly recognized condition that has become a major cause of esophageal symptoms in children and adults. The epidemiology of EoE has been described from multiple countries throughout the world. The frequencies reported in the literature vary depending on the method of data collection and whether cases were identified via registries or population databases, which likely represent a more accurate estimation of the true incidence and prevalence. Although an increase in awareness certainly has contributed to the higher frequencies reported, recent population-based studies suggest that the incidence and prevalence appear to be increasing. The incidence is currently estimated to be approximately 10 cases/100,000 persons annually, whereas the prevalence is reported between 10 and 57 cases/100,000 persons. An increase in awareness of this condition will likely contribute to more cases being diagnosed, and because EoE is a chronic condition, the prevalence is expected to increase as well.

**REFERENCES**

1. Landres RT, Kuster GG, Strum WB. Eosinophilic esophagitis in a patient with vigorous achalasia. Gastroenterology 1978;74(6):1298–301.
2. Dellon ES, Gonsalves N, Hirano I, et al. ACG clinical guideline: evidenced based approach to the diagnosis and management of esophageal eosinophilia and eosinophilic esophagitis (EoE). Am J Gastroenterol 2013;108(5):679–92 [quiz: 693].
3. Moawad FJ, Cheng E, Schoepfer A, et al. Eosinophilic esophagitis: current perspectives from diagnosis to management. Ann N Y Acad Sci 2016;1380(1): 204–17.
4. Dellon ES. Epidemiology of eosinophilic esophagitis. Gastroenterol Clin North Am 2014;43(2):201–18.
5. Syed AA, Andrews CN, Shaffer E, et al. The rising incidence of eosinophilic oesophagitis is associated with increasing biopsy rates: a population-based study. Aliment Pharmacol Ther 2012;36(10):950–8.
6. Dellon ES, Erichsen R, Baron JA, et al. The increasing incidence and prevalence of eosinophilic oesophagitis outpaces changes in endoscopic and biopsy practice: national population-based estimates from Denmark. Aliment Pharmacol Ther 2015;41(7):662–70.
7. Hruz P, Straumann A, Bussmann C, et al. Escalating incidence of eosinophilic esophagitis: a 20-year prospective, population-based study in Olten County, Switzerland. J Allergy Clin Immunol 2011;128(6):1349–50.e5.
8. Dalby K, Nielsen RG, Kruse-Andersen S, et al. Eosinophilic oesophagitis in infants and children in the region of southern Denmark: a prospective study of prevalence and clinical presentation. J Pediatr Gastroenterol Nutr 2010;51(3): 280–2.
9. Giriens B, Yan P, Safroneeva E, et al. Escalating incidence of eosinophilic esophagitis in Canton of Vaud, Switzerland, 1993-2013: a population-based study. Allergy 2015;70(12):1633–9.
10. van Rhijn BD, Verheij J, Smout AJ, et al. Rapidly increasing incidence of eosinophilic esophagitis in a large cohort. Neurogastroenterol Motil 2013;25(1): 47–52.e5.
11. Arias A, Lucendo AJ. Prevalence of eosinophilic oesophagitis in adult patients in a central region of Spain. Eur J Gastroenterol Hepatol 2013;25(2):208–12.
12. Homan M, Blagus R, Jeverica AK, et al. Pediatric eosinophilic esophagitis in slovenia: data from a retrospective 2005-2012 epidemiological study. J Pediatr Gastroenterol Nutr 2015;61(3):313–8.
13. Noel RJ, Putnam PE, Rothenberg ME. Eosinophilic esophagitis. N Engl J Med 2004;351(9):940–1.
14. Prasad GA, Alexander JA, Schleck CD, et al. Epidemiology of eosinophilic esophagitis over three decades in Olmsted County, Minnesota. Clin Gastroenterol Hepatol 2009;7(10):1055–61.
15. Ally MR, Maydonovitch CL, Betteridge JD, et al. Prevalence of eosinophilic esophagitis in a United States military health-care population. Dis Esophagus 2015;28(6):505–11.
16. Dellon ES, Jensen ET, Martin CF, et al. Prevalence of eosinophilic esophagitis in the United States. Clin Gastroenterol Hepatol 2014;12(4):589–96.e1.
17. Gill R, Durst P, Rewalt M, et al. Eosinophilic esophagitis disease in children from West Virginia: a review of the last decade (1995-2004). Am J Gastroenterol 2007; 102(10):2281–5.

18. Murray IA, Joyce S, Palmer J, et al. Incidence and features of eosinophilic esophagitis in dysphagia: a prospective observational study. Scand J Gastroenterol 2016;51(3):257–62.

19. Sperry SL, Crockett SD, Miller CB, et al. Esophageal foreign-body impactions: epidemiology, time trends, and the impact of the increasing prevalence of eosinophilic esophagitis. Gastrointest Endosc 2011;74(5):985–91.

20. Diniz LO, Towbin AJ. Causes of esophageal food bolus impaction in the pediatric population. Dig Dis Sci 2012;57(3):690–3.

21. Gretarsdottir HM, Jonasson JG, Bjornsson ES. Etiology and management of esophageal food impaction: a population based study. Scand J Gastroenterol 2015;50(5):513–8.

22. Kidambi T, Toto E, Ho N, et al. Temporal trends in the relative prevalence of dysphagia etiologies from 1999-2009. World J Gastroenterol 2012;18(32):4335–41.

23. Veerappan GR, Perry JL, Duncan TJ, et al. Prevalence of eosinophilic esophagitis in an adult population undergoing upper endoscopy: a prospective study. Clin Gastroenterol Hepatol 2009;7(4):420–6, 426.e1-2.

24. Joo MK, Park JJ, Kim SH, et al. Prevalence and endoscopic features of eosinophilic esophagitis in patients with esophageal or upper gastrointestinal symptoms. J Dig Dis 2012;13(6):296–303.

25. Sealock RJ, Kramer JR, Verstovsek G, et al. The prevalence of oesophageal eosinophilia and eosinophilic oesophagitis: a prospective study in unselected patients presenting to endoscopy. Aliment Pharmacol Ther 2013;37(8):825–32.

26. Altun R, Akbas E, Yildirim AE, et al. Frequency of eosinophilic esophagitis in patients with esophageal symptoms: a single-center Turkish experience. Dis Esophagus 2013;26(8):776–81.

27. Moawad FJ, Dellon ES, Achem SR, et al. Effects of race and sex on features of eosinophilic esophagitis. Clin Gastroenterol Hepatol 2016;14(1):23–30.

28. De la Cruz-Patino E, Ruiz Juarez I, Meixueiro Daza A, et al. Eosinophilic esophagitis prevalence in an adult population undergoing upper endoscopy in southeastern Mexico. Dis Esophagus 2015;28(6):524–9.

29. Shi YN, Sun SJ, Xiong LS, et al. Prevalence, clinical manifestations and endoscopic features of eosinophilic esophagitis: a pathological review in China. J Dig Dis 2012;13(6):304–9.

30. Fujishiro H, Amano Y, Kushiyama Y, et al. Eosinophilic esophagitis investigated by upper gastrointestinal endoscopy in Japanese patients. J Gastroenterol 2011;46(9):1142–4.

31. Shoda T, Morita H, Nomura I, et al. Comparison of gene expression profiles in eosinophilic esophagitis (EoE) between Japan and Western countries. Allergol Int 2015;64(3):260–5.

32. Kinoshita Y, Ishimura N, Oshima N, et al. Systematic review: eosinophilic esophagitis in Asian countries. World J Gastroenterol 2015;21(27):8433–40.

33. Foroutan M, Norouzi A, Molaei M, et al. Eosinophilic esophagitis in patients with refractory gastroesophageal reflux disease. Dig Dis Sci 2010;55(1):28–31.

34. Sa CC, Kishi HS, Silva-Werneck AL, et al. Eosinophilic esophagitis in patients with typical gastroesophageal reflux disease symptoms refractory to proton pump inhibitor. Clinics (Sao Paulo) 2011;66(4):557–61.

35. Ramakrishnan R, Chong H. Eosinophilic oesophagitis in adults. Histopathology 2008;52(7):897–900.

36. Garcia-Compean D, Gonzalez Gonzalez JA, Marrufo Garcia CA, et al. Prevalence of eosinophilic esophagitis in patients with refractory gastroesophageal reflux disease symptoms: a prospective study. Dig Liver Dis 2011;43(3):204–8.

37. Prasad GA, Talley NJ, Romero Y, et al. Prevalence and predictive factors of eosinophilic esophagitis in patients presenting with dysphagia: a prospective study. Am J Gastroenterol 2007;102(12):2627–32.

38. Mackenzie SH, Go M, Chadwick B, et al. Eosinophilic oesophagitis in patients presenting with dysphagia–a prospective analysis. Aliment Pharmacol Ther 2008;28(9):1140–6.

39. Ricker J, McNear S, Cassidy T, et al. Routine screening for eosinophilic esophagitis in patients presenting with dysphagia. Therap Adv Gastroenterol 2011;4(1): 27–35.

40. Dellon ES, Speck O, Woodward K, et al. Clinical and endoscopic characteristics do not reliably differentiate PPI-responsive esophageal eosinophilia and eosinophilic esophagitis in patients undergoing upper endoscopy: a prospective cohort study. Am J Gastroenterol 2013;108(12):1854–60.

41. Desai TK, Stecevic V, Chang CH, et al. Association of eosinophilic inflammation with esophageal food impaction in adults. Gastrointest Endosc 2005;61(7): 795–801.

42. Kerlin P, Jones D, Remedios M, et al. Prevalence of eosinophilic esophagitis in adults with food bolus obstruction of the esophagus. J Clin Gastroenterol 2007; 41(4):356–61.

43. Hurtado CW, Furuta GT, Kramer RE. Etiology of esophageal food impactions in children. J Pediatr Gastroenterol Nutr 2011;52(1):43–6.

44. Truskaite K, Dlugosz A. Prevalence of eosinophilic esophagitis and lymphocytic esophagitis in adults with esophageal food bolus impaction. Gastroenterol Res Pract 2016;2016:9303858.

45. Cherian S, Smith NM, Forbes DA. Rapidly increasing prevalence of eosinophilic oesophagitis in Western Australia. Arch Dis Child 2006;91(12):1000–4.

46. Mansoor E, Cooper GS. The 2010-2015 prevalence of eosinophilic esophagitis in the USA: a population-based study. Dig Dis Sci 2016;61(10):2928–34.

47. Maradey-Romero C, Prakash R, Lewis S, et al. The 2011-2014 prevalence of eosinophilic oesophagitis in the elderly amongst 10 million patients in the United States. Aliment Pharmacol Ther 2015;41(10):1016–22.

48. Spergel JM, Book WM, Mays E, et al. Variation in prevalence, diagnostic criteria, and initial management options for eosinophilic gastrointestinal diseases in the United States. J Pediatr Gastroenterol Nutr 2011;52(3):300–6.

49. Kim S, Kim S, Sheikh J. Prevalence of eosinophilic esophagitis in a population-based cohort from Southern California. J Allergy Clin Immunol Pract 2015;3(6): 978–9.

50. Ronkainen J, Talley NJ, Aro P, et al. Prevalence of oesophageal eosinophils and eosinophilic oesophagitis in adults: the population-based Kalixanda study. Gut 2007;56(5):615–20.

51. Abonia JP, Wen T, Stucke EM, et al. High prevalence of eosinophilic esophagitis in patients with inherited connective tissue disorders. J Allergy Clin Immunol 2013;132(2):378–86.

52. Thompson JS, Lebwohl B, Reilly NR, et al. Increased incidence of eosinophilic esophagitis in children and adults with celiac disease. J Clin Gastroenterol 2012;46(1):e6–11.

53. Stewart MJ, Shaffer E, Urbanski SJ, et al. The association between celiac disease and eosinophilic esophagitis in children and adults. BMC Gastroenterol 2013;13:96.
54. Peterson K, Firszt R, Fang J, et al. Risk of autoimmunity in EoE and families: a population-based cohort study. Am J Gastroenterol 2016;111(7):926–32.
55. Davis BP, Epstein T, Kottyan L, et al. Association of eosinophilic esophagitis and hypertrophic cardiomyopathy. J Allergy Clin Immunol 2016;137(3):934–6.e5.
56. Hurrell JM, Genta RM, Dellon ES. Prevalence of esophageal eosinophilia varies by climate zone in the United States. Am J Gastroenterol 2012;107(5):698–706.
57. Almansa C, Krishna M, Buchner AM, et al. Seasonal distribution in newly diagnosed cases of eosinophilic esophagitis in adults. Am J Gastroenterol 2009;104(4):828–33.
58. Moawad FJ, Veerappan GR, Lake JM, et al. Correlation between eosinophilic oesophagitis and aeroallergens. Aliment Pharmacol Ther 2010;31(4):509–15.

# Demographic Features of Eosinophilic Esophagitis

Anna Maria Lipowska, MD[a], Robert T. Kavitt, MD, MPH[b],*

## KEYWORDS

- Eosinophilic esophagitis • Demographics • Epidemiology • Dysphagia

## KEY POINTS

- Eosinophilic esophagitis affects both pediatric and adult patients, with most patients being Caucasian men.
- Most studies on eosinophilic esophagitis have been performed in the Western world.
- Certain populations, such as African Americans and women, may be underdiagnosed because of their presentation with atypical symptoms.

## INTRODUCTION

Eosinophilic esophagitis (EoE) is an increasingly prevalent chronic condition characterized by eosinophilic infiltration of the esophageal epithelium accompanied by esophageal symptoms. The number of new diagnoses is growing worldwide in both pediatric and adult populations.[1–4] Differences in disease distribution and presentation have been found, varying by gender, race, and other characteristics. This review aims to examine the existing literature and to provide insight into the demographic features of EoE.

## AGE

EoE affects both children and adults and can present with a variety of symptoms depending on age. An examination of children with EoE around the world demonstrated similar demographics to adult cases, noting the presence of concomitant atopic disease as well as a male predominance.[5–7] Adults are most commonly diagnosed in young adulthood, in their third decade of life.[8]

In rare cases, new EoE diagnoses are made in the elderly as well.[9] A case report noted an 89-year-old man presenting with new dysphagia symptoms and in whom

Disclosure Statement: The authors have nothing to disclose.
[a] Section of Gastroenterology, Hepatology, and Nutrition, The University of Chicago Medicine, 5841 South Maryland Avenue, MC 4076, Room M421, Chicago, IL 60637, USA; [b] Center for Esophageal Diseases, Section of Gastroenterology, Hepatology, and Nutrition, The University of Chicago Medicine, 5841 South Maryland Avenue, MC 4080, Chicago, IL 60637, USA
* Corresponding author.
E-mail address: rkavitt@medicine.bsd.uchicago.edu

a diagnosis of EoE was confirmed endoscopically and by histology, highlighting that physicians should maintain a wide differential in all patients.[10] Furthermore, a large nationwide study found that 7.6% of patients with EoE are aged 65 years or older.[11] This subset of older patients had a higher likelihood of gastroesophageal reflux disease and was less likely to be male. Of note, this population is also less commonly diagnosed with concurrent asthma and food allergies.

The most typical symptom among adults at the time of diagnosis is dysphagia, which contrasts with presenting symptoms of children and adolescents.[12,13] Infants and toddlers with eosinophilic gastrointestinal disease most frequently present with feeding dysfunction.[14] As children age, they instead experience vomiting, gastroesophageal reflux, and abdominal pain, and once they reach their teenage years dysphagia is most commonly reported.[15,16] The underlying cause of this shift in presenting symptoms is thought to be a progression from inflammatory esophageal changes to fibrotic remodeling.[17] Out of all the presenting symptoms in childhood, dysphagia has the highest likelihood to persist into adulthood.[18] However, childhood EoE symptoms do not always last with time. A recent prospective study found that 81% of patients diagnosed with EoE in childhood experience resolution or regression of their symptoms as young adults.[18]

Aside from symptoms, data regarding differences in histologic features between pediatric and adult EoE patients are limited.[13] In a large nationwide study, no significant differences were found between age groups in peak mucosal eosinophil count.[9]

## GENDER

In both children and adults, men are more frequently diagnosed with EoE than women. Studies have estimated that EoE patients are 2 to 3 times more likely to be male than female.[9,19,20] A recent meta-analysis evaluated the prevalence ratio by gender, finding a pooled prevalence for male patients of 53.8 per 100,000 inhabitants compared with 20.1 for female patients.[21]

To date, little research has been performed investigating gender-based differences in EoE. Lynch and colleagues[22] executed a case-controlled study comparing the initial EoE presentation between men and women. Interestingly, women more commonly presented with heartburn, whereas men more commonly presented with dysphagia or a food impaction. These trends may suggest that fibrostenotic disease characterized by esophageal remodeling and deposition of subepithelial fibrosis may be more likely in men than women, or that women are more likely to experience the inflammatory component of EoE. Similar findings of predominant dysphagia symptoms in male patients were found by Sperry and colleagues,[23] although neither study observed endoscopic differences between the sexes. In addition, no differences between men and women were observed in histologic features and frequency of atopic disease.

## RACE

EoE has a 3-fold higher prevalence among Caucasian patients compared with other races.[24] Studies have shown that between 84% and 95% of EoE patients are Caucasian.[15,25] A population-based study in the United States published in 2016 assessing more than 7000 patients with EoE found that 89.3% were Caucasian, 6.1% were African American, and 5.6% were Asian.[26]

A comparison of Caucasian, African American, and Hispanic patients found that Caucasians were more likely to experience dysphagia symptoms and have abnormal findings on endoscopy, but no difference was found on histology among the groups.[27]

Esophageal rings on endoscopy were also more common in Caucasians, whereas African Americans were more likely to have normal-appearing esophageal mucosa.[23] Overall, evidence suggests that African American patients with EoE may be underdiagnosed given less typical symptoms and more subtle or absent endoscopic findings.

Surprisingly, many studies of children affected by EoE do not describe race data. One study found that a significantly larger percentage of EoE pediatric patients are non-white compared with adults.[28] African American children are diagnosed at a younger age and are less likely to present with dysphagia.[28,29] On biopsy, mean mid-esophageal eosinophil count was found to be higher in African American children.[29] When adjusted for Caucasian race, socioeconomic status was not found to be associated with diagnosis of EoE in children and adolescents.[25]

## GEOGRAPHY

Most studies regarding EoE have emerged from Western countries, with data limited from other parts of the world. An examination of EoE prevalence in China estimated that the disease affects 0.4% of the adult population.[30] A review of EoE in Asian countries incorporating 25 articles and 217 patients found a similar proportion of men (73%) to studies of predominantly Caucasian patients.[31] Another comparison of Caucasian and Asian EoE patients revealed a similar ratio of 70% men and 30% women.[32]

Compared with Caucasians, research suggests that Asians are more likely to experience vomiting and abdominal pain and less likely to present with dysphagia and heartburn.[32] However, conflicting data exist, with another study suggesting that dysphagia was the most commonly reported symptom, similar to Caucasian patients.[31] Notably, this study identified food impactions in less than 5% of patients with EoE in Asian countries. Likewise, a report comparing Asian and Western populations confirmed food impactions to be a strikingly rare occurrence in Asians.[33] Many patients had a history of allergic diseases, with EoE most frequently associated with bronchial asthma.[31]

Even less is known about EoE in Latin America. A small study of 150 patients with refractory gastroesophageal reflux disease in Mexico demonstrated that 4% of this patient population received a diagnosis of EoE.[34] A more recent study of Mexican mestizos undergoing elective endoscopy found an EoE prevalence of 1.7%.[35]

In the United States, no clear regional predisposition to higher EoE prevalence has been defined. A large study of the US military health care population found an increased EoE prevalence in the western region of the country as well as in the northern states.[19] On the other hand, a survey study of physicians found that EoE was more likely to be present in the northeastern United States and in the urban setting.[36]

## CLIMATE

Given that environmental factors are thought to play a role in EoE pathogenesis, investigators have scrutinized geographic location and climate differences as a potential key to improving the understanding of EoE. Research suggests that cold and arid climates may be associated with esophageal eosinophilia. A large study of patients in the United States found an elevated odds ratio of 1.39 for cold latitudes and an odds ratio of 1.27 for arid climates.[37] The odds of esophageal eosinophilia were not significantly higher for patients in tropical climates.

Furthermore, seasonal variation has not been found to be convincingly associated with frequency of EoE diagnosis and EoE flares. Although some studies have demonstrated a positive association between season and diagnosis of EoE, they do not account for the duration of symptoms preceding diagnosis. A meta-analysis of newly recognized EoE cases demonstrated an even distribution of new diagnoses throughout the year.[38] This study also did not find variation in food impaction incidence between the seasons. Similarly, a large retrospective cohort study confirmed an even distribution year round of food bolus obstruction events.[39]

## ASSOCIATED DISORDERS

EoE has been found to be associated with atopic diseases, including bronchial asthma, atopic dermatitis, rhinitis, and food allergies.[13] A study of an EoE patient cohort found that more than three-quarters of patients had at least one atopic disease. In this group, the prevalence of asthma was 39.0%, allergic rhinitis 61.9%, and atopic dermatitis 46.1%, all higher than in the general population.[40] A systematic review and meta-analysis also confirmed that asthma, allergic rhinitis, and eczema were all more significantly common among EoE patients than among controls.[41] An examination of IgE-mediated food allergies in pediatric patients found a higher prevalence of EoE in this population compared with the general population.[42]

Aside from atopic disorders, EoE has been associated with multiple other conditions. A variety of studies have described a link between EoE and inflammatory bowel disease, connective tissue disease, esophageal atresia, and celiac disease, among other conditions. Proliferation of gastrointestinal eosinophils leading to worsening gut inflammation is commonly seen in inflammatory bowel disease. Individual reports have described an association between the 2 disease states, although large studies are needed to confirm dependence.[43,44] Individuals with connective tissue disease have been found to have an 8-fold risk of having EoE.[45] A potential association has also been noted between EoE and esophageal atresia patients, particularly in those with persistent dysphagia and refractory reflux symptoms.[46–48]

Findings have been mixed with respect to an association between celiac disease and EoE.[49–51] The trend was more visible in pediatric patients; however, data remain limited.[52] A large population-based study of adult patients found that EoE patients had no increased risk of celiac disease.[53] A more recent systematic review and meta-analysis also supported this finding.[54,55]

## SUMMARY

Further investigation is needed into EoE demographics to promote a better understanding of the disease. EoE has been found to predominantly affect Caucasians; however, studies suggest that other populations including African Americans may be underdiagnosed because of presentation with atypical symptoms. Men are more frequently diagnosed with EoE than women, yet men are also more likely to present with classic dysphagia symptoms, whereas the only symptom some female patients with EoE experience is heartburn. Geographic trends suggest an association with urban environments and possibly colder climates. However, data regarding these subjects are limited, and more research needs to be performed worldwide to thoroughly investigate trends in EoE prevalence, demographics, endoscopic and histologic characteristics, and treatment response.

## REFERENCES

1. Hruz P, Straumann A, Bussmann C, et al. Escalating incidence of eosinophilic esophagitis: a 20-year prospective, population-based study in Olten County, Switzerland. J Allergy Clin Immunol 2011;128(6):1349–50.e5.

2. Prasad GA, Alexander JA, Schleck CD, et al. Epidemiology of eosinophilic esophagitis over three decades in Olmsted County, Minnesota. Clin Gastroenterol Hepatol 2009;7(10):1055–61.

3. Straumann A, Simon HU. Eosinophilic esophagitis: escalating epidemiology? J Allergy Clin Immunol 2005;115(2):418–9.

4. Soon IS, Butzner JD, Kaplan GG, et al. Incidence and prevalence of eosinophilic esophagitis in children. J Pediatr Gastroenterol Nutr 2013;57(1):72–80.

5. Homan M, Blagus R, Jeverica AK, et al. Pediatric eosinophilic esophagitis in Slovenia: data from a retrospective 2005-2012 epidemiological study. J Pediatr Gastroenterol Nutr 2015;61(3):313–8.

6. Gomez Torrijos E, Sanchez Miranda P, Donado Palencia P, et al. Eosinophilic esophagitis: demographic, clinical, endoscopic, histologic, and atopic characteristics of children and teenagers in a region in Central Spain. J Investig Allergol Clin Immunol 2017;27(2):104–10.

7. Assiri AM, Saeed A. Incidence and diagnostic features of eosinophilic esophagitis in a group of children with dysphagia and gastroesophageal reflux disease. Saudi Med J 2014;35(3):292–7.

8. Croese J, Fairley SK, Masson JW, et al. Clinical and endoscopic features of eosinophilic esophagitis in adults. Gastrointest Endosc 2003;58(4):516–22.

9. Kapel RC, Miller JK, Torres C, et al. Eosinophilic esophagitis: a prevalent disease in the United States that affects all age groups. Gastroenterology 2008;134(5):1316–21.

10. Trifan A, Stoica O, Chihaia CA, et al. Eosinophilic esophagitis in an octogenarian: a case report and review of the literature. Medicine (Baltimore) 2016;95(41):e5169.

11. Maradey-Romero C, Prakash R, Lewis S, et al. The 2011-2014 prevalence of eosinophilic oesophagitis in the elderly amongst 10 million patients in the United States. Aliment Pharmacol Ther 2015;41(10):1016–22.

12. Straumann A, Aceves SS, Blanchard C, et al. Pediatric and adult eosinophilic esophagitis: similarities and differences. Allergy 2012;67(4):477–90.

13. Lucendo AJ, Sanchez-Cazalilla M. Adult versus pediatric eosinophilic esophagitis: important differences and similarities for the clinician to understand. Expert Rev Clin Immunol 2012;8(8):733–45.

14. Mukkada VA, Haas A, Maune NC, et al. Feeding dysfunction in children with eosinophilic gastrointestinal diseases. Pediatrics 2010;126(3):e672–7.

15. Assa'ad AH, Putnam PE, Collins MH, et al. Pediatric patients with eosinophilic esophagitis: an 8-year follow-up. J Allergy Clin Immunol 2007;119(3):731–8.

16. Noel RJ, Putnam PE, Rothenberg ME. Eosinophilic esophagitis. N Engl J Med 2004;351(9):940–1.

17. Dellon ES, Kim HP, Sperry SL, et al. A phenotypic analysis shows that eosinophilic esophagitis is a progressive fibrostenotic disease. Gastrointest Endosc 2014;79(4):577–85.e4.

18. Bohm M, Jacobs JW Jr, Gupta A, et al. Most children with eosinophilic esophagitis have a favorable outcome as young adults. Dis Esophagus 2017;30(1):1–6.

19. Ally MR, Maydonovitch CL, Betteridge JD, et al. Prevalence of eosinophilic esophagitis in a United States military health-care population. Dis Esophagus 2015;28(6):505–11.

20. Furuta GT, Liacouras CA, Collins MH, et al. Eosinophilic esophagitis in children and adults: a systematic review and consensus recommendations for diagnosis and treatment. Gastroenterology 2007;133(4):1342–63.

21. Arias A, Perez-Martinez I, Tenias JM, et al. Systematic review with meta-analysis: the incidence and prevalence of eosinophilic oesophagitis in children and adults in population-based studies. Aliment Pharmacol Ther 2016;43(1):3–15.
22. Lynch KL, Dhalla S, Chedid V, et al. Gender is a determinative factor in the initial clinical presentation of eosinophilic esophagitis. Dis Esophagus 2016;29(2): 174–8.
23. Sperry SL, Woosley JT, Shaheen NJ, et al. Influence of race and gender on the presentation of eosinophilic esophagitis. Am J Gastroenterol 2012;107(2): 215–21.
24. Hruz P. Epidemiology of eosinophilic esophagitis. Dig Dis 2014;32(1–2):40–7.
25. Franciosi JP, Tam V, Liacouras CA, et al. A case-control study of sociodemographic and geographic characteristics of 335 children with eosinophilic esophagitis. Clin Gastroenterol Hepatol 2009;7(4):415–9.
26. Mansoor E, Cooper GS. The 2010-2015 prevalence of eosinophilic esophagitis in the USA: a population-based study. Dig Dis Sci 2016;61(10):2928–34.
27. Bohm M, Malik Z, Sebastiano C, et al. Mucosal eosinophilia: prevalence and racial/ethnic differences in symptoms and endoscopic findings in adults over 10 years in an urban hospital. J Clin Gastroenterol 2012;46(7):567–74.
28. Weiler T, Mikhail I, Singal A, et al. Racial differences in the clinical presentation of pediatric eosinophilic esophagitis. J Allergy Clin Immunol Pract 2014;2(3):320–5.
29. Gill RK, Al-Subu A, Elitsur Y, et al. Prevalence and characteristics of eosinophilic esophagitis in 2 ethnically distinct pediatric populations. J Allergy Clin Immunol 2014;133(2):576–7.
30. Ma X, Xu Q, Zheng Y, et al. Prevalence of esophageal eosinophilia and eosinophilic esophagitis in adults: a population-based endoscopic study in Shanghai, China. Dig Dis Sci 2015;60(6):1716–23.
31. Kinoshita Y, Ishimura N, Oshima N, et al. Systematic review: eosinophilic esophagitis in Asian countries. World J Gastroenterol 2015;21(27):8433–40.
32. Ito J, Fujiwara T, Kojima R, et al. Racial differences in eosinophilic gastrointestinal disorders among Caucasian and Asian. Allergol Int 2015;64(3):253–9.
33. Ishimura N, Shimura S, Jiao D, et al. Clinical features of eosinophilic esophagitis: differences between Asian and Western populations. J Gastroenterol Hepatol 2015;30(Suppl 1):71–7.
34. Garcia-Compean D, Gonzalez Gonzalez JA, Marrufo Garcia CA, et al. Prevalence of eosinophilic esophagitis in patients with refractory gastroesophageal reflux disease symptoms: a prospective study. Dig Liver Dis 2011;43(3):204–8.
35. De la Cruz-Patino E, Ruiz Juarez I, Meixueiro Daza A, et al. Eosinophilic esophagitis prevalence in an adult population undergoing upper endoscopy in southeastern Mexico. Dis Esophagus 2015;28(6):524–9.
36. Spergel JM, Book WM, Mays E, et al. Variation in prevalence, diagnostic criteria, and initial management options for eosinophilic gastrointestinal diseases in the United States. J Pediatr Gastroenterol Nutr 2011;52(3):300–6.
37. Hurrell JM, Genta RM, Dellon ES. Prevalence of esophageal eosinophilia varies by climate zone in the United States. Am J Gastroenterol 2012;107(5):698–706.
38. Lucendo AJ, Arias A, Redondo-Gonzalez O, et al. Seasonal distribution of initial diagnosis and clinical recrudescence of eosinophilic esophagitis: a systematic review and meta-analysis. Allergy 2015;70(12):1640–50.
39. Philpott HL, Nandurkar S, Thien F, et al. Seasonal recurrence of food bolus obstruction in eosinophilic esophagitis. Intern Med J 2015;45(9):939–43.

40. Mohammad AA, Wu SZ, Ibrahim O, et al. Prevalence of atopic comorbidities in eosinophilic esophagitis: a case-control study of 449 patients. J Am Acad Dermatol 2017;76(3):559–60.
41. Gonzalez-Cervera J, Arias A, Redondo-Gonzalez O, et al. Association between atopic manifestations and eosinophilic esophagitis: a systematic review and meta-analysis. Ann Allergy Asthma Immunol 2017;118(5):582–90.e2.
42. Hill DA, Dudley JW, Spergel JM. The prevalence of eosinophilic esophagitis in pediatric patients with IgE-mediated food allergy. J Allergy Clin Immunol Pract 2017; 5(2):369–75.
43. Mulder DJ, Hookey LC, Hurlbut DJ, et al. Impact of Crohn disease on eosinophilic esophagitis: evidence for an altered T(H)1-T(H)2 immune response. J Pediatr Gastroenterol Nutr 2011;53(2):213–5.
44. Suttor VP, Chow C, Turner I. Eosinophilic esophagitis with Crohn's disease: a new association or overlapping immune-mediated enteropathy? Am J Gastroenterol 2009;104(3):794–5.
45. Abonia JP, Wen T, Stucke EM, et al. High prevalence of eosinophilic esophagitis in patients with inherited connective tissue disorders. J Allergy Clin Immunol 2013;132(2):378–86.
46. Krishnan U. Eosinophilic esophagitis in children with esophageal atresia. Eur J Pediatr Surg 2015;25(4):336–44.
47. Dhaliwal J, Tobias V, Sugo E, et al. Eosinophilic esophagitis in children with esophageal atresia. Dis Esophagus 2014;27(4):340–7.
48. Chan LJ, Tan L, Dhaliwal J, et al. Treatment outcomes for eosinophilic esophagitis in children with esophageal atresia. Dis Esophagus 2016;29(6):563–71.
49. Thompson JS, Lebwohl B, Reilly NR, et al. Increased incidence of eosinophilic esophagitis in children and adults with celiac disease. J Clin Gastroenterol 2012;46(1):e6–11.
50. Jensen ET, Eluri S, Lebwohl B, et al. Increased risk of esophageal eosinophilia and eosinophilic esophagitis in patients with active celiac disease on biopsy. Clin Gastroenterol Hepatol 2015;13(8):1426–31.
51. Ahmed OI, Qasem SA, Abdulsattar JA, et al. Esophageal eosinophilia in pediatric patients with celiac disease: is it a causal or an incidental association? J Pediatr Gastroenterol Nutr 2015;60(4):493–7.
52. Stewart MJ, Shaffer E, Urbanski SJ, et al. The association between celiac disease and eosinophilic esophagitis in children and adults. BMC Gastroenterol 2013;13:96.
53. Ludvigsson JF, Aro P, Walker MM, et al. Celiac disease, eosinophilic esophagitis and gastroesophageal reflux disease, an adult population-based study. Scand J Gastroenterol 2013;48(7):808–14.
54. Hommeida S, Alsawas M, Murad MH, et al. The association between celiac disease and eosinophilic esophagitis: mayo experience and meta-analysis of the literature. J Pediatr Gastroenterol Nutr 2017;65(1):58–63.
55. Lucendo AJ, Arias A, Tenias JM. Systematic review: the association between eosinophilic oesophagitis and coeliac disease. Aliment Pharmacol Ther 2014; 40(5):422–34.

# Latest Insights on the Relationship Between Symptoms and Biologic Findings in Adults with Eosinophilic Esophagitis

Ekaterina Safroneeva, PhD[a],*, Alex Straumann, MD[b,c], Alain M. Schoepfer, MD[d]

## KEYWORDS

- Eosinophilic esophagitis • Patient-reported outcomes • Symptoms • Quality of life
- Regulatory authorities

## KEY POINTS

- Earlier studies had conflicting results on the nature of the relationship between symptoms and biologic findings.
- Based on studies using newly validated PRO measures, the relationship between symptoms and biologic findings in adult patients with EoE is of a nonlinear nature: symptoms tend to be indicative of severe biologic alterations, but lack of symptoms does not exclude presence of mild to moderate biologic alterations.

*Continued*

Disclaimers: None.
Conflict of Interest: E. Safroneeva received consulting fees from Aptalis Pharma, Inc, and Novartis, AG, Switzerland. A. Straumann received consulting fees and/or speaker fees and/or research grants from Actelion, AG, Switzerland, AstraZeneca, AG, Switzerland, Aptalis Pharma, Inc, Dr. Falk Pharma, GmbH, Germany, Glaxo Smith Kline, AG, Nestlé S. A., Switzerland, Novartis, AG, Switzerland, Pfizer, AG, and Regeneron Pharmaceuticals. A. Schoepfer received consulting fees and/or speaker fees and/or research grants from Adare Pharmaceuticals, Inc, AstraZeneca, AG, Switzerland, Aptalis Pharma, Inc, Dr. Falk Pharma, GmbH, Germany, Glaxo Smith Kline, AG, Nestlé S. A., Switzerland, Receptos, Inc, and Regeneron Pharmaceuticals.
Writing Assistance: None.
Grant Support: This work was supported by a grant from the Swiss National Science Foundation (grant no. 32473B_160115), a grant from TIGERS (The International Gastrointestinal Eosinophil ResearcherS), and CEGIR (Consortium of EGID Researchers).
<sup>a</sup> Institute of Social and Preventive Medicine, University of Bern, Finkenhubelweg 11, Bern, 3012, Switzerland; <sup>b</sup> EoE Center, Praxis Römerhof, Römerstrasse 7, Olten, 4600, Switzerland; <sup>c</sup> Division of Gastroenterology and Hepatology, University Hospital Zurich, Rämistrasse 100, Zurich, 8006, Switzerland; <sup>d</sup> Division of Gastroenterology and Hepatology, Centre Hospitalier Universitaire Vaudois, Rue du Bugnon 44, Lausanne, 1011, Switzerland
* Corresponding author.
*E-mail address:* ekaterina.safroneeva@ispm.unibe.ch

Gastrointest Endoscopy Clin N Am 28 (2018) 35–45
http://dx.doi.org/10.1016/j.giec.2017.08.001

*Continued*

- This nonlinear relationship between symptoms and biologic findings has important implications for length of diagnostic delay, selection of the patients for the trials and observational studies, and long-term management of patients with EoE.

## INTRODUCTION

Eosinophilic esophagitis (EoE) is defined as a chronic, immune/antigen-mediated, esophageal disease, characterized clinically by symptoms related to esophageal dysfunction and histologically by eosinophil-predominant inflammation. Adults typically present with swallowing- and nonswallowing-associated pain and dysphagia for solid food that is accompanied by a range of behaviors associated with these symptoms.[1,2] Children, however, experience an array of symptoms, such as vomiting, abdominal pain, and dysphagia, but these seem to vary with age and can be nonspecific.[1,2]

## THE TALE OF TWO STUDIES AND NONLINEAR RELATIONSHIP BETWEEN SYMPTOMS AND BIOLOGIC FINDINGS

Literature often highlights the controversial relationship between biologic findings and symptoms in adult patients with EoE. For example, Straumann and colleagues[3] have demonstrated in a randomized, placebo-controlled 15-day trial of adult/adolescent patients (36 patients, 18 patients in the experimental group, mean esophageal eosinophil count at baseline of 148 [standard deviation ± 61] per high-power field [hpf]) that treatment with topical budesonide improved histologic findings and symptoms as assessed by an ad hoc–developed patient-reported outcomes (PROs) instrument designed to assess dysphagia frequency and severity of dysphagia episodes (Straumann Dysphagia Instrument). However, in a randomized, placebo-controlled 6-week trial of 42 adult patients with mean esophageal eosinophil count at baseline of 26 (range, 12–89 per hpf), Alexander and colleagues[4] showed that treatment with topical fluticasone improves the esophageal eosinophilia, but not symptoms as assessed by two items of the Mayo Dysphagia Questionnaire 14-day version (validated but not specifically for EoE PRO instrument).

In light of the current literature, it is absolutely clear that these studies epitomize two pieces of puzzle that, when put together, tell a great deal about "the controversial" relationship between symptoms and biologic findings. However, without the data from larger observational studies (discussed later), patient selection for the studies is found to be somewhat challenging. In fact, researchers grappling with any condition for which no disease-specific validated PRO measures have been developed have faced similar challenges. For example, using the data of a much larger trial that compared three types of treatment (infliximab alone, azathioprine alone, and combined treatment with infliximab and azathioprine in 508 patients), Peyrin-Biroulet and colleagues[5] have shown an apparent "disconnect" between the biologic disease activity as assessed by systemic C-reactive protein, fecal calprotectin levels, and clinical activity as assessed by Crohn's Disease Activity Index (CDAI). CDAI is a composite measure that includes, among other things, clinician-reported symptoms, laboratory findings, and presence of complications. Authors attributed such disconnect to CDAI properties, namely lack of specificity of included symptoms for the diseases and lack of sensitivity of these symptoms for inflammation observed during colonoscopy. In the era before US Food and Drug Administration (FDA) guidance for PRO development, inflammatory bowel disease (IBD) researchers might have included nonspecific and systemic symptoms into the clinical activity measure; however, inclusion of nonspecific symptoms, albeit assessed by nonvalidated instruments, as end points in adult trials is less relevant to the EoE field because dysphagia, the main symptom in this patient population, is organ specific.[6] As such, lack of disease-specific symptoms in adult trials cannot explain this disconnect between symptoms and biologic findings in adult EoE.

This brings us to the second point about the sensitivity of symptoms in detecting inflammation and fibrosis, another hallmark of this disease. In ulcerative colitis, elevated calprotectin levels precede the development of symptoms indicative of flare by 3 months.[7] At the moment, lack of noninvasive laboratory markers precludes EoE researchers from obtaining that type of data. With the Cytosponge (PA Consulting Group, Melbourn, UK), esophageal string test, and quantification of eosinophil degranulation urinary 3-bromotyrosine levels on the way, such data may soon shine a light on this topic in measuring more sensitive markers of active inflammation.[8–10] However, in the absence of these tools, there are other ways of looking at this symptom-inflammation disconnect. One such way is by examining the relationship between symptoms and epithelial findings using data on large groups of patients with various degrees of biologic severity and symptoms (either in the context of therapy trials or cross-sectional observational studies).

Until recently most trials and even observational studies were small, and symptoms were often assessed either retrospectively, as simple dichotomous outcome, or using nonvalidated or non-disease-specific instruments, which precluded the easy interpretation of the findings. In 2014, however, the EoE esophagitis community came together to develop a PRO measure as a part of the EoE Activity Index study (EEsAI), during which endoscopic, histologic, and symptom data on 270 patients were collected prospectively.[11] These more recent data clearly point to the fact that adult symptoms, such as frequency of dysphagia, various behavioral adaptations to living with this condition, and swallowing-associated pain, indeed correlate with biologic findings and are indicative of severe inflammatory and fibrotic alterations. For example, individuals with severe rings, intermediate-to-high-grade strictures, severe exudates, and peak eosinophil counts greater than 320 eosinophils/mm$^2$ (roughly >100 per hpf) are likely to experience the kind of symptom severity that differs drastically from patients in whom these features are either absent or present in mild/moderate form and eosinophil counts less than or equal to 100 per hpf. This relationship between EEsAI PRO and biologic disease severity is mirrored by the relationship between EoE-specific quality of life as assessed by Adult Eosinophilic Esophagitis Quality of Life instrument and biologic findings.[12]

Along a similar vein, when Chen and colleagues[13] examined the relationship between esophageal distensibility as assessed by functional luminal imaging probe and symptoms, they observed that all adult patients with severe rings were likely to have a history of food impaction when compared with 20%, 25%, and 39% in patients with absent, mild, or moderate rings, respectively. The authors were not able to show that severe inflammation impacts the esophageal distensibility or is associated with history of food impaction, but the number of subjects with severe exudates was fairly low in that study. If one looks at symptom severity in patients with absence of endoscopic or histologic findings, it is nearly identical to that of patients with mild endoscopic and histologic alterations. When using the data on severity of adult patients' symptoms and biologic findings collected in the course of EEsAI study, we and other collaborators observed that symptom score of 20 points (range, 0–100 points) had modest accuracy in identifying patients in endoscopic and histologic remission (little over 60%).[14] EoE symptoms correlate with endoscopic and histologic activity; however, their negative predictive value is insufficient (**Fig. 1**).

Another important point that is often brought up in the context of this "controversial" relationship between symptoms and biologic findings in EoE is related to the limited ability to assess esophageal fibrotic alterations in routine studies, as functional luminal imaging probe technology undergoes further evolution and is not used universally. It is often argued that this vital technology may explain away some of the controversy. However, because individuals on the low end of biologic severity spectrum have little to no symptoms, it is highly unlikely that one will be able to explain apparent lack of symptoms with this extra bit of knowledge about the biologic alterations in this disease. As such, just as in IBD, the sensitivity of EoE symptoms in detecting inflammation and fibrosis seems to be limited, and the relationship between mucosal inflammation, fibrosis, and symptoms/EoE-specific quality of life as assessed by PRO measures is nonlinear.

The nonlinear nature of the relationship between symptoms and biologic findings in adult EoE has implications for, among other things, the timing of diagnosis in relation to appearance of symptoms, patient selection, PROs use, placebo effect in the interventional studies, and long-term care of patients with EoE (discussed later).

## DIAGNOSTIC DELAY IN EOSINOPHILIC ESOPHAGITIS

Given that low grades of esophageal inflammation can be asymptomatic yet lead to fibrosis, it is not surprising that patients with mild esophageal inflammation or fibrosis might not experience the kind of symptoms that urge the patients to seek immediate medical help. Furthermore, these findings are consistent with a long diagnostic delay, defined as time from symptom onset to the time of diagnosis, typically observed in adults with EoE. For example, adult patients with EoE in Switzerland are diagnosed after a median delay of 6 years.[15] The mild to moderate biologic alterations that do not readily translate into perceptible symptoms as observed in the patient is one of the factors that contribute to this long diagnostic delay in EoE patients. However, other

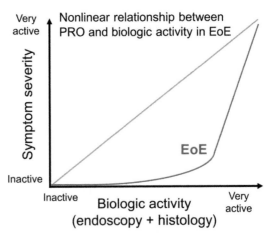

**Fig. 1.** Eosinophilic esophagitis is characterized by a nonlinear relationship between PRO and endoscopic and histologic activity. Such a nonlinear relationship between PRO and biologic activity is also observed in other diseases, such as Crohn disease, ulcerative colitis, and asthma.

factors, such as the fact that patients might exercise behavioral adaptations to ease living with dysphagia and mitigate the severity of this symptom, the hidden nature of the affected organ, and the relative low prevalence of this condition (and hence less than optimal awareness among physicians) contribute to long diagnostic delays in EoE.[16,17] As patients, gastroenterologists, and general practitioners become more aware of EoE, it is likely that the diagnostic delay will decrease. Nevertheless, in the absence of a routinely assessed and readily available biologic marker, such delay will likely never be as short as that for other inflammatory disorders, such as Crohn disease (diagnostic delay of 5–9 months), or those with external manifestations that patients can observe, such as joint swelling in inflammatory rheumatic diseases (diagnostic delay of 3–4 months).[18,19]

## IMPLICATIONS FOR FUTURE TRIALS

The previously mentioned studies about the nonlinear relationship between symptoms and biologic severity have important implications for trial design in adult EoE.

For many diseases presenting with characteristic symptoms and biologic alterations, the FDA clearly advocates for the use of coprimary end points with symptoms and biologic alterations being assessed as outcomes. This type of end point ensures that patients with symptoms have objective signs of disease-specific alterations (and the other way around) and that improvement in the degree of severity of these alterations corresponds to the improvement in disease-specific symptoms. To be able to demonstrate a meaningful improvement in adult patients with EoE, care should be taken to enroll patients with fairly severe and/or frequent symptoms (eg, EEsAI PRO score >50) that are likely to manifest themselves in the presence of obvious endoscopic and histologic alterations, both inflammatory and fibrotic in nature. However, if the medication is expected to have mostly an anti-inflammatory effect and is tested in a short trial, the patients with fairly severe fibrotic alterations, such as intermediate- to high-grade strictures, should be excluded from the trial because symptoms caused by strictures in these individuals are not likely to improve over a short period of time.

In recent years, several studies evaluating the efficacy of different formulations of budesonide and monoclonal therapy with anti-interleukin (IL)-13 examined symptom and quality of life improvement in adult and adolescent patients with EoE using validated or newly developed EoE-specific PRO symptom and quality of life measures, such as the Dysphagia Symptom Questionnaire (DSQ), Daily Symptom Diary (DSD), EEsAI, and Adult Eosinophilic Esophagitis Quality of Life.[11,20–22] Some of these instruments have been described and extensively reviewed with respect to the presence of important measurement properties that would affect their applicability, whereas little information is available on measures that are currently undergoing validation, such as DSD.[23,24] The symptom-specific PRO measures have 24-hour recall period (7-day recall is also available for EEsAI) and assess the frequency and/or severity of dysphagia, although swallowing-associated pain and behavioral adaptations to living with dysphagia are also assessed by some of these measures.

Use of these instruments combined with the better understanding of the nonlinear nature of the relationship between biologic findings and symptoms in EoE, lead to recruitment of patients with more severe biologic alterations and symptoms into these trials to more likely achieve symptom response. Although two of these studies have only been published in an abstract form, only patients with mean eosinophil counts of more than 70 eosinophils per hpf presumably reflecting a more severe inflammatory phenotype of the disease were recruited to all these studies. For example, in a randomized, double-blind, placebo-controlled study of monoclonal anti-IL-13 antibody (RPC4046), patients received either 180 mg of RPC4046 (n = 31), 360 mg of RPC4046 (n = 34), or placebo (n = 34). The baseline peak esophageal eosinophil count ranged from 92 to 123 per hpf and was reduced significantly in the groups treated with the drug but not with the placebo.[19] Although this study was not powered to assess symptom improvement and was fairly small, a trend toward improvement in DSD was observed in patients treated with a higher dose of this medication. Similarly, in a randomized, double-blind, placebo-controlled study by Lucendo and colleagues,[25] authors used budesonide orodispersible tablet (1 mg twice daily; n = 59) or placebo (n = 29) for 6-week treatment of adult patients with EoE. budesonide orodispersible tablet, 1 mg twice daily, was highly statistically superior to placebo in achieving clinicohistologic remission (57.6% vs 0%; P<.001), histologic remission (93.2% vs 0%; P<.001), clinical remission (59.3% vs 13.8%; P<.001), and endoscopic remission (61.0% vs 0%; P<.001). A prolonged treatment of up to 12 weeks increased the overall cumulative clinicohistologic remission rate up to 84.7%. This study should remind us not to expect a significant symptom improvement in most of the treated patients in the first couple of weeks but to give some time to judge symptom improvement (**Fig. 2**).

Lastly, in a double-blind, randomized, placebo-controlled study by Dellon and colleagues,[26] adult and adolescent patients with EoE were treated with 2 mg of budesonide oral suspension twice daily for a period of 12 weeks (87 patients, 49 in the budesonide group, mean esophageal eosinophil count at baseline of 156.3 [standard deviation ± 98] per hpf). A validated PROs symptom measure, the DSQ, was used as coprimary end point. DSQ is a daily diary with the score ranging from 0 to 84 points (when examined over a 2-week period; higher scores indicate more frequent and severe dysphagia episodes). A significant difference in DSQ score decrease (of 14.3 points when compared with 7.5 points in placebo group) and esophageal eosinophilia drop were observed when patients treated with budesonide were compared with those treated with placebo. To summarize, use of new-generation validated instruments in these types of trials leads to a fairly consistent improvement in severity of biologic alterations and symptoms (albeit modest), even when all studies were small, if patients with at least moderate gross and microscopic EoE are studied.

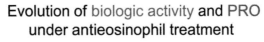

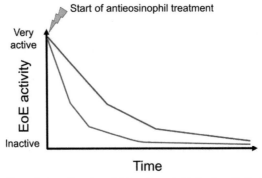

**Fig. 2.** On introduction of an antieosinophil treatment, biologic activity (endoscopy and histology) tends to improve quicker than symptoms. Thus, clinical studies should evaluate PRO for a sufficient amount of time if PRO improvement is targeted as a study endpoint.

When one closely examines the studies in other fields, such as asthma, the improvement observed in symptoms in patients treated with drug when compared with those treated with placebo as assessed by PRO instruments including the five-item Asthma Control Questionnaire (score ranges from 0 to 6 points), St. George's Respiratory Questionnaire (score ranges from 0 to 100 points), or 22-item Sinonasal Outcome Test is often modest and also dependent on the degree of underlying inflammation. For example, in a study examining the efficacy of mepolizumab (anti-IL-5) in patients with severe asthma (and recurrent exacerbations; n = 576), a difference in St. George's Respiratory Questionnaire score change from baseline to end of treatment of 6.4 and 7 points (a drop of four points was considered to be clinically relevant) was observed between two drug-treated arms and placebo was observed.[27] In a study of dupilumab (antibody to the alpha subunit of the IL-4 receptor) in patients with persistent asthma (n = 104), an improvement of 0.73 points (0.5 points is the minimal clinically important difference) over placebo was observed.[28] As such, it seems that the kind of symptom responses that are observed in adult EoE trials are consistent with those in other internal allergic diseases, such as asthma, where there is a broad range of fibrosis and inflammation.

Although the use of comprehensive PRO symptom instruments, especially those with daily recall, seems to be a hallmark of many new therapy trials in adult EoE, it is also important to point out that the use of simpler tools, such as visual analog scales and 10-point Likert scales, has been shown to be effective in detecting response to treatment in clinical trials and observational studies or examining symptom variation in a cross-sectional study.[11,19,23,29] In fact, score derivation for EEsAI PRO was carried out using patient global assessment of symptom severity as gold standard.

Another unique trait of the budesonide oral suspension efficacy study, when looking at all adult trials in EoE, is a 4-week placebo run-in period used to ensure that patients with too few episodes of dysphagia did not enter the main part of the study. However, it was also interesting to learn that 24 of 93 patients had greater than or equal to 30% decrease in DSQ score (defined as symptom response) during this period.[30] In a randomized, double-blind, placebo-controlled study by Miehlke and colleagues[31] the authors used budesonide orodispersible tablet (1 mg twice daily, and 2 mg twice daily) and viscous suspension (2 mg twice daily) for 2-week treatment of adult patients with EoE. Although most patients treated with various formulations of budesonide achieved histologic remission (baseline peak esophageal eosinophil count of more than 200 per $mm^2$ of hpf), more than 95% of all patients treated with budesonide achieved histologic remission of less than 16 eosinophils per $mm^2$ of hpf. These patients had a symptom response as assessed by nonvalidated Straumann Dysphagia Instrument that was indistinguishable from that in patients treated with placebo. It seems that in the first month of treatment, a fairly substantial symptom improvement is observed in patients treated with placebo effect.

These data are reminiscent of the kind of placebo effects observed in asthma and IBD studies, when PRO and clinician-reported instruments, respectively, are used to assess symptoms and disease-specific quality of life. For example, in the already mentioned mepolizumab trial, a profound drop in Asthma Control Questionnaire-5 (about 0.4 points) was observed not only with drug but also in placebo-treated patients (mirrored by increase in forced expiratory volume in 1 second, which to some extent depends on patient compliance).[25] In a trial of vedolizumab (anti $\alpha_4\beta_7$ integrin antibody), a drop in CDAI of roughly 50 points occurred in all the study groups, including placebo, for the first 30 weeks of the study (response was defined as drop of $\geq$100 points).[32] As more is learned about EoE-specific PRO instruments and more EoE trials are conducted (including those with placebo run-in periods), it will be learned whether longer trial periods are needed to demonstrate a symptom response to therapy, as is the case in many other fields. It also needs to be understood better if a placebo response is purely symptomatic or biologic.

## LONG-TERM MANAGEMENT OF EOSINOPHILIC ESOPHAGITIS

Just as patients may sustain a histologic response in the absence of symptom resolution, a lack of symptoms does not indicate lack of inflammatory and fibrotic alterations. As a result, such patients cannot be followed based on symptoms and should undergo esophagogastroduodenoscopy to monitor biologic findings. In addition, physicians seeing the patients with this disease face the ultimate challenge: encouraging patients with asymptomatic EoE with subclinical esophageal inflammation to continue their anti-inflammatory pharmacologic therapy. However, the question arises whether physicians should encourage the patients to undergo follow-up and continue their therapy in the absence of symptoms. The answer is: yes. The retrospective analyses of the data from groups of patients from Switzerland and United States have shown that duration of diagnostic delay is positively associated with formation of fibrotic alterations, such as rings and strictures, that in the long-term cause most symptoms and are risk factors for food-bolus impactions.[15,33]

Furthermore, a recent study by Greuter and colleagues[34] showed that 82% of adult patients that achieved long-lasting ($\geq$6 months) clinical, endoscopic, and histologic remission following median 89 weeks of treatment with swallowed topical corticosteroids, experienced clinical relapse after a median 22 weeks off therapy. Although this is a first study of its kind, many of the previously mentioned compounds will also be evaluated in the long-term maintenance trials, which will undoubtedly shed more light on this topic. Nevertheless, EoE physicians would have to borrow a page or two from studies on untreated hypertension, diabetes, and other chronic conditions, and conduct studies on how to best motivate patients in self-reported good to excellent health to adhere to therapy given the inevitable recurrence of disease once therapy is stopped.

## SUMMARY (OR TWO STUDIES REVISITED)

So what can be learned from the two studies that have triggered this major controversy of symptoms versus histology in adult EoE? Looking closely at the studies by Straumann and colleagues[3] and Alexander and colleagues,[4] it is absolutely clear that with markedly elevated baseline eosinophilia of 135 eosinophils per hpf (>439 eosinophils/mm$^2$), the Swiss study was much more likely to be defined by a patient population with severe rings, strictures, exudates, and more importantly a high enough number of dysphagia episodes per week to detect symptomatic and histologic improvement, when compared with the Mayo Clinic study, into which patients with mild inflammation were recruited. Alexander and colleagues[4] showed that patients with 26 eosinophils per hpf (83–102 eosinophils/mm$^2$) are likely to have mild to no symptoms that could be improved in a meaningful way and therefore lack evidence of symptom to histology correlation.

The results of these studies provided the first evidence for the nonlinear nature of the relationship between symptoms and biologic findings in adults with EoE depending on the degree of underlying mucosal inflammation. This has important implications for the diagnosis, patient selection for the trials, and long-term management of this condition. Patients with EoE are likely to be diagnosed with a delay that is in part attributed to the lack of profound symptoms in the presence of mild biologic alterations. When selecting subjects for the trials, care should be taken to recruit individuals with at least moderately severe biologic alterations and symptoms to show a meaningful improvement. The use of validated PRO measures and simple numeric scales to assess symptoms and disease-specific quality of life in these trials is encouraged. The symptom improvement observed in most recent trials is modest (and most likely clinically meaningful) and consistent with modest symptom improvement observed in trials of other chronic conditions, such as asthma or IBD. The trials should be at least 6 to 8 weeks long given the symptom improvement on placebo in the first month of the trial. The lack of symptoms at low biologic severity disease spectrum introduces the need for the follow-up that included esophagogastroduodenoscopy, and presents physicians with a challenge of encouraging asymptomatic patients to adhere to therapy.

As one looks into the future of symptom assessment in EoE, it is absolutely crucial that clinicians continue to validate the PRO measures; develop definitions of response and remission; and improve their properties by, among other things, making better use of various quantitative methods to support PRO development, such as classical test theory early in the PRO development and item response theory in later stages, because this may require fairly large sample sizes.[35] Many of the PRO developers out of necessity, low patient numbers, and time considerations, examine a single symptom of EoE: dysphagia. Although this symptom is not at all easy to assess, one may hope for the tools that begin with incorporate quite a few symptoms of this disease, undergo item reduction, and score derivations based on these more labor-intensive methods. Development of these types of measure requires the kind concerted efforts between research community and pharmaceutical industry attempted by Evidera's Exacerbations of Chronic Pulmonary Disease Tool PRO Initiative, which resulted in the development of the first FDA-approved PRO measure.[36]

## REFERENCES

1. Dellon ES, Gonsalves N, Hirano I, et al. ACG clinical guideline: evidenced based approach to the diagnosis and management of esophageal eosinophilia and eosinophilic esophagitis (EoE). Am J Gastroenterol 2013;108:679–92.

2. Lucendo AJ, Molina-Infante J, Arias A, et al. Guidelines on eosinophilic esophagitis: evidence-based statements and recommendations for diagnosis and management in children and adults. United Eur Gastroenterol J 2017;5:335–58.

3. Straumann A, Conus S, Degen L, et al. Budesonide is effective in adolescent and adult patients with active eosinophilic esophagitis. Gastroenterology 2010;139: 1526–37.

4. Alexander JA, Jung KW, Arora AS, et al. Swallowed fluticasone improves histologic but not symptomatic response of adults with eosinophilic esophagitis. Clin Gastroenterol Hepatol 2012;10:742–9.

5. Peyrin-Biroulet L, Reinisch W, Colombel JF, et al. Clinical disease activity, C-reactive protein normalisation and mucosal healing in Crohn's disease in the SONIC trial. Gut 2014;63:88–95.

6. Guidance for industry patient-reported outcome measures: use in medical product development to support labeling claims. U.S. Food and Drug Administration. Available at: https://www.fda.gov/downloads/drugs/guidances/ucm193282.pdf. Accessed September 6, 2017.

7. De Vos M, Louis EJ, Jahnsen J, et al. Consecutive fecal calprotectin measurements to predict relapse in patients with ulcerative colitis receiving infliximab maintenance therapy. Inflamm Bowel Dis 2013;19:2111–7.

8. Katzka DA, Geno DM, Ravi A, et al. Accuracy, safety, and tolerability of tissue collection by Cytosponge vs endoscopy for evaluation of eosinophilic esophagitis. Clin Gastroenterol Hepatol 2015;13:77–83.

9. Fillon SA, Harris JK, Wagner BD, et al. Novel device to sample the esophageal microbiome: the esophageal string test. PLoS One 2012;7:e42938.

10. Cunnion KM, Willis LK, Minto HB, et al. Eosinophil quantitated urine kinetic: a novel assay for assessment of eosinophilic esophagitis. Ann Allergy Asthma Immunol 2016;116:435–9.

11. Schoepfer AM, Straumann A, Panczak R, et al. Development and validation of a symptom-based activity index for adults with eosinophilic esophagitis. Gastroenterology 2014;147:1255–66.

12. Safroneeva E, Coslovsky M, Kuehni CE, et al. Eosinophilic oesophagitis: relationship of quality of life with clinical, endoscopic and histological activity. Aliment Pharmacol Ther 2015;42:1000–10.

13. Chen JW, Pandolfino JE, Lin Z, et al. Severity of endoscopically identified esophageal rings correlates with reduced esophageal distensibility in eosinophilic esophagitis. Endoscopy 2016;48:794–801.

14. Safroneeva E, Straumann A, Coslovsky M, et al. Symptoms have modest accuracy in detecting endoscopic and histologic remission in adults with eosinophilic esophagitis. Gastroenterology 2016;150:581–90.

15. Schoepfer AM, Safroneeva E, Bussmann C, et al. Delay in diagnosis of eosinophilic esophagitis increases risk for stricture formation in a time-dependent manner. Gastroenterology 2013;145:1230–6.

16. Giriens B, Yan P, Safroneeva E, et al. Escalating incidence of eosinophilic esophagitis in Canton of Vaud, Switzerland, 1993-2013: a population-based study. Allergy 2015;70:1633–9.

17. Hruz P, Straumann A, Bussmann C, et al. Escalating incidence of eosinophilic esophagitis: a 20-year prospective, population-based study in Olten County, Switzerland. J Allergy Clin Immunol 2011;128:1349–50.

18. Vavricka SR, Spigaglia SM, Rogler G, et al. Systematic evaluation of risk factors for diagnostic delay in inflammatory bowel disease. Inflamm Bowel Dis 2012;18:496–505.

19. Sørensen J, Hetland ML, All Departments of Rheumatology in Denmark. Diagnostic delay in patients with rheumatoid arthritis, psoriatic arthritis and ankylosing spondylitis: results from the Danish nationwide DANBIO registry. Ann Rheum Dis 2015;74:e12.

20. Dellon ES, Irani AM, Hill MR, et al. Development and field testing of a novel patient-reported outcome measure of dysphagia in patients with eosinophilic esophagitis. Aliment Pharmacol Ther 2013;38:634–42.

21. Hirano I, Collins MH, Assouline-Dayane Y, et al. A randomized, double-blind, placebo-controlled trial of novel recombinant, humanized, anti-interleukin-13 monoclonal antibody (RPC4046) in patients with active eosinophilic esophagitis: results of the heroes study. United Eur Gastroenterol J 2016;2(Supplement 1).

22. Taft TH, Kern E, Kwiatek MA, et al. The adult eosinophilic oesophagitis quality of life questionnaire: a new measure of health-related quality of life. Aliment Pharmacol Ther 2011;34:790–8.

23. Schoepfer A, Safroneeva E, Straumann A. How to measure disease activity in eosinophilic esophagitis. Dis Esophagus 2016;29:959–66.

24. Patel DA, Sharda R, Hovis KL, et al. Patient-reported outcome measures in dysphagia: a systematic review of instrument development and validation. Dis Esophagus 2017;30:1–23.

25. Lucendo A, Miehlke S, Vieth M, et al. Budesonide orodispersible tablets are highly effective for treatment of active eosinophilic esophagitis: results from a randomized, double-blind, placebo-controlled, pivotal multicenter trial (EOS-1). Gastroenterology 2017;152:S207.
26. Dellon ES, Katzka DA, Collins MH, et al. Budesonide oral suspension improves symptomatic, endoscopic, and histologic parameters compared with placebo in patients with eosinophilic esophagitis. Gastroenterology 2017;152:776–86.
27. Ortega HG, Liu MC, Pavord ID, et al. Mepolizumab treatment in patients with severe eosinophilic asthma. N Engl J Med 2014;371:1198–207.
28. Beck LA, Thaçi D, Hamilton JD, et al. Dupilumab treatment in adults with moderate-to-severe atopic dermatitis. N Engl J Med 2014;371:130–9.
29. Reed CC, Wolf WA, Cotton CC, et al. A visual analogue scale and a Likert scale are simple and responsive tools for assessing dysphagia in eosinophilic oesophagitis. Aliment Pharmacol Ther 2017;45:1443–8.
30. Hirano I, Williams J, Collins MH, et al. Clinical features at baseline are not clearly associated with symptomatic placebo response in adolescents and adults with eosinophilic esophagitis during a placebo run-in period of a double-blind, randomized, controlled trial of budesonide oral suspension. Gastroenterology 2017;152:S854.
31. Miehlke S, Hruz P, Vieth M, et al. A randomised, double-blind trial comparing budesonide formulations and dosages for short-term treatment of eosinophilic oesophagitis. Gut 2016;65:390–9.
32. Sandborn WJ, Brian G, Feagan BG, et al. Vedolizumab as induction and maintenance therapy for Crohn's disease. N Engl J Med 2013;369:711–21.
33. Lipka S, Kumar A, Richter JE. Impact of diagnostic delay and other risk factors on eosinophilic esophagitis phenotype and esophageal diameter. J Clin Gastroenterol 2016;50:134–40.
34. Greuter T, Bussmann C, Safroneeva E, et al. Long-term treatment of eosinophilic esophagitis with swallowed topical corticosteroids: development and evaluation of a therapeutic concept. Am J Gastroenterol 2017. [Epub ahead of print].
35. Cappelleri JC, Jason Lundy J, Hays RD. Overview of classical test theory and item response theory for the quantitative assessment of items in developing patient-reported outcomes measures. Clin Ther 2014;36:648–62.
36. Leidy NK, Murray LT, Monz BU, et al. Measuring respiratory symptoms of COPD: performance of the EXACT- Respiratory Symptoms Tool (E-RS) in three clinical trials. Respir Res 2014;15:124.

# Endoscopic and Radiologic Findings in Eosinophilic Esophagitis

Jeffrey A. Alexander, MD, FACP

## KEYWORDS

- Eosinophilic esophagitis • Endoscopic findings EoE • Radiographic findings EoE
- Endoscopic reflux score • Barium esophagram

## KEY POINTS

- Endoscopic findings of exudates, rings, furrows, edema, and stricture are frequently seen in eosinophilic esophagitis (EoE).
- These findings are not completely specific for the diagnosis.
- An endoscopic reflux score can be calculated from these findings and correlates with disease activity, but does not alleviate the need for histologic sampling.
- A barium esophagram can show rings, strictures, and small-caliber esophagus in EoE.
- Barium esophagram is a more sensitive test at evaluating esophageal diameter than endoscopy.

## ENDOSCOPIC FINDINGS

In general, the endoscopic findings of eosinophilic esophagitis (EoE) are highly suggestive but not diagnostic of the disease.[1] The findings can be seen in the entire esophagus or in isolated segments of the esophagus. Not infrequently, these findings may be seen in the more proximal esophagus. Endoscopic findings are not completely sensitive or specific for the diagnosis. Most publications on EoE present highly selected studies. In studies looking at less selected patients undergoing upper gastrointestinal endoscopy (EGD) and routine biopsy, eosinophilic esophageal inflammation (>20 eosinophils [eos] per high-power field [hpf]) was present in 12% of unselected adult patients with dysphagia,[2] in 15% of adult patients with dysphagia without another evident cause,[3] and in 6.5% of adult patients undergoing EGD for any reason.[4] In these studies, 16% to 33% of these adult EoE patients had no endoscopic findings of the disease.[2,3] Similarly, the specificity of endoscopic findings is

Disclosures: The author has financial interest in Meritage Pharmacia/Shire Pharmaceutical.
Division of Gastroenterology and Hepatology, Mayo Clinic School of Medicine, 200 First Street Southwest, Rochester, MN 55905, USA
E-mail address: alexander.jeffrey14@mayo.edu

incomplete. These studies were remarkably similar in that only 34% to 40% of the patients with endoscopic rings were found to have significant esophageal eosinophilia.[2–4] It was suggested early in the EoE story, that the lack of sensitivity of endoscopic findings was a result of underrecognition,[5] but as experience with the disease has progressed, the endoscopically normal esophagus in a minority of EoE patients has persisted.[6–8]

The field moved forward significantly with the publication of a standardized and validated reference system for EoE findings published by Hirano and colleagues[9] in 2013. These findings can be used to calculate the eosinophilic esophagitis endoscopic reference score (EREFS): exudates, rings, edema, furrows, and strictures. The EREFS classification allowed clinicians and investigators to have a standard terminology and a standard scoring system for the endoscopic findings of EoE for clinical practice and trials, respectively.

### Major Features

### Exudates

Exudates are whitish plaques in the esophagus that are thought to represent eosinophilic inflammation. These plaques can easily be misinterpreted as candidiasis. Exudates are classified as grade 1, mild: lesions taking up less than 10% of the esophageal mucosa, and 2, severe: taking up greater than 10% of the esophageal mucosa (**Fig. 1**).[9] Exudates are a finding that was not well described in the earlier descriptions of EoE. In a meta-analysis of 100 studies involving 4678 patients, Kim and colleagues[10] found the sensitivity and specificity of exudates in EoE were 27% and 94%, respectively.

### Rings

Rings can be one to several millimeters thick and easily recognized endoscopically (**Fig. 2**). Rings must persist with esophageal air insufflation. Ringlike structures that deflate with air insufflation are termed feline esophagus. This term had been used often in early descriptions of EoE but was poorly defined. It is likely many of the earlier studies in EoE did not differentiate feline esophagus from fixed esophageal rings that persist with air insufflation. The author suspects in clinical practices there remains some imprecision in the use of this term. Therefore, the sensitivity and specificity of feline esophagus in the diagnosis of EoE are uncertain.

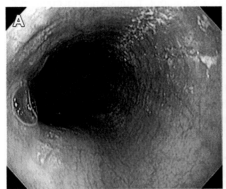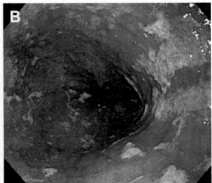

**Fig. 1.** Classification of exudates. (*A*) *Grade 1*: White lesions involving <10% of the surface area of the esophagus. (*B*) *Grade 2*: White lesions involving >10% of the surface area of the esophagus. (*From* Hirano I, Moy N, Heckman MG, et al. Endoscopic assessment of the oesophageal features of eosinophilic oesophagitis: validation of a novel classification and grading system. Gut 2013;62:489–95; with permission.)

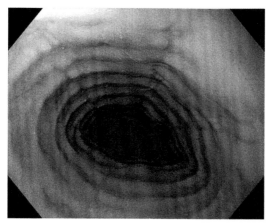

**Fig. 2.** Typical rings with furrows.

Rings in the esophagus are classified as grade 1, mild: subtle circumferential ridges; grade 2, moderate: distinct rings that do not impair the passage of a standard upper endoscope (8–10 mm); and grade 3, severe: distinct rings that do not permit passage of the standard endoscope (**Fig. 3**).[9] Kim and colleagues[10] found the pooled sensitivity and specificity of rings for EoE to be 48% and 91%, respectively. Of note, in most of these studies, selected patients were reported. The specificity of endoscopic rings was significantly lower in studies wherein endoscopy was performed in unselected patients. As mentioned above, 20 eos/hpf were found in only 40% or less of less selected patients with endoscopic rings present.[2–4]

*Edema*
Edema is defined as the loss of vascular pattern and can be manifest as a generalized mucosal pallor. Edema is present or absent and is classified as grade 1, loss of clarity or absence of vascular markings (**Fig. 4**).[9] The presence or absence is only described in the minority of EoE studies. The sensitivity and specificity of edema for EoE are 43% and 90%, respectively.[10]

*Furrows*
Longitudinal furrows are likely the most common finding in EoE. They are typically seen as long linear lines with some subtle irregularities that run parallel up and

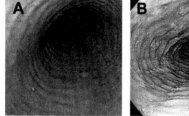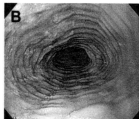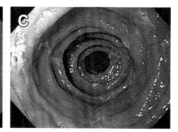

**Fig. 3.** Classification of rings. (*A*) *Grade 1*: Subtle circumferential ridges seen during esophageal distension. (*B*) *Grade 2*: Distinct rings that do not occlude passage of standard adult diagnostic. (*C*) *Grade 3*: Distinct rings that do not permit passage of standard adult diagnostic endoscope. (*From* Hirano I, Moy N, Heckman MG, et al. Endoscopic assessment of the oesophageal features of eosinophilic oesophagitis: validation of a novel classification and grading system. Gut 2013;62:489–95; with permission.)

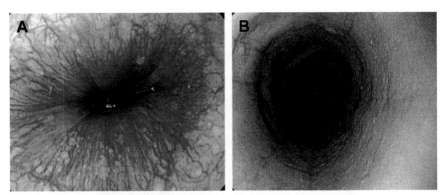

**Fig. 4.** Classification of edema. (*A*) *Grade 0*: Distinct vascular markings. (*B*) *Grade 1*: Loss of clarity or absence of vascular markings. (*From* Hirano I, Moy N, Heckman MG, et al. Endoscopic assessment of the oesophageal features of eosinophilic oesophagitis: validation of a novel classification and grading system. Gut 2013;62:489–95; with permission.)

down the esophagus. They appear as confined breaks in the mucosa (which is what they likely are). They have also been termed train tracks and longitudinal markings. These furrows, similar to rings, must persist with esophageal air insufflation. They are classified as grade 1, mild: vertical lines without depth, and grade 2, severe: with mucosal depth (**Fig. 5**).[9] The sensitivity and specificity of furrows for EoE were 40% and 95%, respectively, in the Kim analysis.[10]

*Stricture*
Strictures related to esophageal remodeling are common in EoE and are classified in the EREFS systems as merely present (grade 1) or absent (grade 0).[9] Others have classified strictures as low-grade (offering some resistance to passing the 9 mm scope), intermediate grade (able to pass the 6-mm scope but not the 9-mm scope), and high grade (unable to pass the 6-mm scope).[11] Fibrotic disease in EoE can be focal (≤1 cm in length), long (several centimeters in length), or present as diffuse small-caliber esophagus taking up most of the esophageal length (**Fig. 6**).[12] Longer

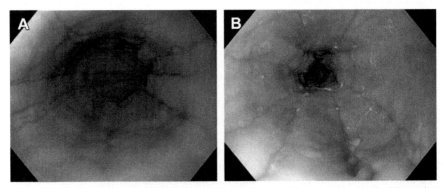

**Fig. 5.** Classification of furrows. (*A*) *Grade 1*: Vertical lines without visible depth. (*B*) *Grade 2*: Vertical lines with visible depth. (*From* Hirano I, Moy N, Heckman MG, et al. Endoscopic assessment of the oesophageal features of eosinophilic oesophagitis: validation of a novel classification and grading system. Gut 2013;62:489–95; with permission.)

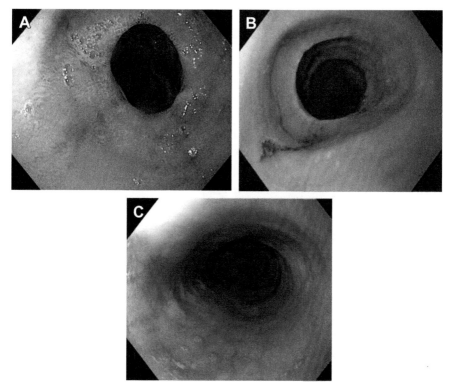

**Fig. 6.** Other Features of EoE. (*A*) Short ring like stricture. (*B*) Long stricture. (*C*) Diffuse small-caliber esophagus. (*From* Hirano I, Moy N, Heckman MG, et al. Endoscopic assessment of the oesophageal features of eosinophilic oesophagitis: validation of a novel classification and grading system. Gut 2013;62:489–95; with permission.)

strictures and small-caliber esophagus can be somewhat difficult to evaluate endoscopically if the luminal diameter is greater than 10 mm. Interobserver agreement of this finding was only moderate in the Hirano study.[9] This diffuse narrowing is better recognized with measurement of esophageal distensibility with the endoflip device or by structured barium esophagram.[12,13]

## Other Features

### Crepe paper esophagus

Crepe paper esophagus, a term used to describe the mucosal fragility seen in EoE, was one of the first recognized endoscopic findings in this disease[5,14] (**Fig. 7A**). Crepe paper esophagus is displayed as significant mucosal injury, sheering or tearing after minimal trauma, including passing the endoscope alone without biopsy or dilation performed.

### Feline esophagus

As mentioned above, feline esophagus is defined as mucosal rings observed during endoscopy that may be more prominent with belching or retching that disappear with air insufflation. Interobserver agreement of feline esophagus is poor, and it is not incorporated into the EREFS.[9] Feline esophagus likely represents transient longitudinal muscle shortening.

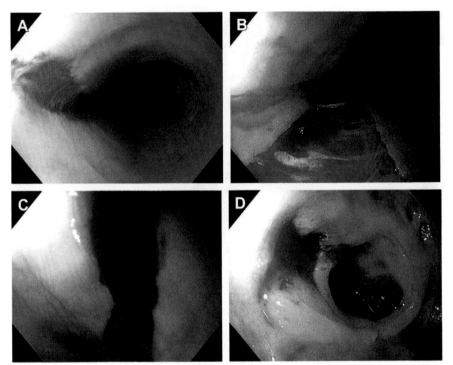

**Fig. 7.** Other features of EoE. (*A*) Crepe paper esophagus. (*B*) Deep mucosal tear post-dilation. (*C*) Deep mucosal tear post-dilation. (*D*) Deep mucosal tear post-dilation of a Schatski Ring. (*From* Hirano I, Moy N, Heckman MG, et al. Endoscopic assessment of the oesophageal features of eosinophilic oesophagitis: validation of a novel classification and grading system. Gut 2013;62:489–95; with permission.)

### Pull sign

This term reflects the sensation of the mucosa feeling firm and offering resistance to pulling the forceps back after it is closed when securing a biopsy specimen. The pull sign was reported in one study to be moderately sensitive and highly specific for EoE.[15]

### Postdilation deep mucosal tears

Deep mucosal tears after esophageal dilation were reported early in the EoE experience.[5,14,16] The deep tears often develop even with minimally traumatic esophageal dilations (see **Fig. 7**B, C). The sensitivity and specificity of this finding for EoE have not been well evaluated. However, in the author's clinical experience, he finds these deep mucosal tears seen after a dilation with mild resistance to be almost pathognominic for EoE. Deep tears such as this from dilation of Schatzki rings in his experience are frequently associated with esophageal eosinophilia rather than gastroesophageal reflux disease (see **Fig. 7**D).

### Normal esophagus

In the meta-analysis by Kim and colleagues,[10] the presence of more than one endoscopic finding of EoE had a sensitivity and specificity of 87% and 47%, respectively for EoE. A normal endoscopic appearance was seen in 17% of patients in the retrospective studies and 7% of patients in prospective studies in that review.[10] Of note, most of these studies in the meta-analysis reflect selected patients. In 2 prospective studies of unselected patients, the prevalence of endoscopically normal EoE was significantly higher. In these studies, in which all patients with dysphagia or dysphagia without other causes were biopsied, 30% to 40% of patients with greater than 20 eos/hpf had normal endoscopies.[2,3] The author suspects using the current cutoff of 15 eos/hpf, and with more experience with the disease, the true incidence of endoscopically normal EoE is likely in the range of 10%.

### Miscellaneous

Furrows, exudates, and edema are thought to represent inflammatory findings. They have been reported to resolve in most patients in some early studies[17,18] but not in others.[19–21] Two recent studies, however, have shown persistent inflammatory findings in most patients in histologic remission.[22] Rings are likely a mixed inflammatory and fibrotic feature. They may resolve in a minority of cases with anti-inflammatory therapy.[7,22,23] Strictures, in general, are more fibrotic and related to esophageal remodeling. In general, they do not resolve with short-term therapy. However, esophageal distensibility may improve somewhat with control of inflammation,[24,25] giving hope that there may be reversibility of fibrosis over time.

Histologic inflammation tends to correlate with areas of endoscopically visualized abnormalities[26]; it seems reasonable to perform biopsies in areas of endoscopic inflammatory changes.

The EREFS Endoscopic Reference Score is scored as the sum of the values as outlined above.[9] The system has moderate to substantial interobserver and intraobserver agreement for endoscopic findings of EoE.[9,23] The EREFS has been shown to be higher in patients with active tissue eosinophilia than those in remission, but the score cannot reliably predict histologic remission.[7,22,23] In attempts to make the EREFS score more clinically useful, a subclassification of EREFS into a fibrotic score (rings and strictures) and an inflammatory score (exudate, furrows, edema) has been proposed.[23] Similarly, Dellon and colleagues[7] have proposed a weighted scoring system by doubling the scores for exudates, rings, and edema. However, at this point in time, histologic esophageal sampling is still required to access response to therapy. Nonetheless, many think the combination of endoscopic and histologic evaluation has clinical value as opposed to reliance on one of these parameters alone.

## RADIOGRAPHIC FINDINGS

Radiographic findings in EoE have received much less attention than endoscopic findings. Radiography is not useful at identifying the inflammatory findings of edema and exudates but can be useful for evaluation of fibrostenotic disease. Fixed rings are commonly seen on barium esophagography. Furthermore, a barium esophagram is more sensitive than endoscopy for the evaluation of an esophageal stricture and diffuse small-caliber esophagus.[12]

The author performs a structured barium esophagram in all his EoE patients. This structured examination has the patient drink barium as fast as possible, and an esophageal image is obtained at maximal esophageal distention. A calculated maximal and minimal diameter is obtained, which needs to be corrected for body habitus. A maximal diameter of ≥20 mm and a minimal diameter of ≥15 are normal.[24] This examination gives not only a baseline of fibrotic disease that helps to determine treatment and prognosis but also a nonendoscopic means of objectively following the disease long term.

## Rings

Fixed rings can be seen radiographically throughout the esophagus or localized to an esophageal segment (**Fig. 8**A). These rings can often appear as "a stack of coins" and are often tightly grouped. Distal rings can be seen in EoE in groups or individually. What relationship the rings in this location have to gastroesophageal reflux disease is uncertain. The Schatzki ring deserves some discussion. In studies where unselected patients with dysphagia were biopsied, 5% to 8% of patients with Schatzki rings had significant esophageal eosinophilia.[2,3] As mentioned above, in the author's experience, deep mucosal tears associated with endoscopically appearing Schatzki rings are often associated with esophageal eosinophilia. These tears may reflect the transmural stricturing associated with this Schatzki ring (indeed, ring is a misnomer in this case). In contrast, those patients with true rings, defined as membranous encircling within the gastroesophageal junction, have gastroesophageal reflux disease. When this narrowing is more stricturelike, the differentiation of reflux from an allergic cause can be difficult.

## Strictures

Esophageal remodeling with subepithelial fibrosis and stricture formation is extremely common in EoE.[11,27–29] This structuring is further supported by loss of esophageal compliance as measured by the Endoflip found commonly in adults with EoE.[13] Radiography is highly accurate at evaluating esophageal strictures associated with EoE. It is a noninvasive, relatively inexpensive, and readily available technology. Esophageal narrowing has been classified by the length of the fixed narrowing as (1) rings ($\leq$1 cm), (2) strictures ($\leq$8 cm), and (3) small-caliber esophagus (>8 cm)[12] (see **Fig. 8**). A structured esophageal examination is a more sensitive technique to evaluate EoE

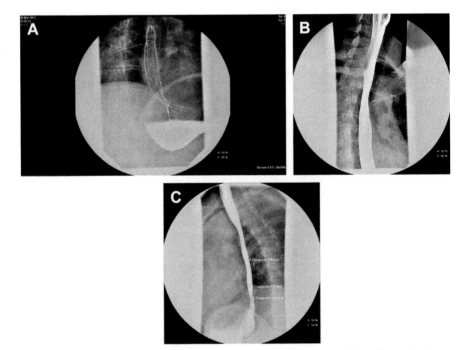

**Fig. 8.** (A) Proximal esophageal rings. (B) Multiple rings forming a midesophageal stricture. (C) Diffuse small-caliber esophagus. Arrow to proximal esophageal rings.

stricturing disease than endoscopy. For example, in patients with an esophageal diameter less than 15 mm on esophagography, less than three-quarters of endoscopic procedures will detect the stricture.[12] For those patients with an esophageal diameter less than 13 mm, only about 24% to 33% of strictures will be detected endoscopically.[12] The challenge in performing barium esophagrams in patients with EoE is identifying a gastrointestinal radiologist willing to perform this type of structured study.

The radiographic study does affect the management of patients. The author is generally more aggressive with the long-term medical or dietary therapy in those with significant esophageal narrowing. Moreover, the esophageal diameter predicts the need for esophageal dilation; in the author's experience, all patients in histologic remission with diameters of ≤10 mm and very few of those with greater than 15 mm will require dilation for symptom relief.[12]

## SUMMARY

Endoscopy in EoE has moved from the recognition of interesting findings to an objective tool with a validated scoring system to more accurately grade the degree of disease. Use of this grading system will become imperative to follow patients and to perform clinical trials. Similarly, barium esophagography has become a complementary test for endoscopy with its increased sensitivity for the diagnosis and characterizations of esophageal strictures in EoE. Independent of histology, these tests have become not only an important means of assessing severity and response to disease but also serve as additional biomarkers of EoE.

## REFERENCES

1. Landres RT, Kuster GG, Strum WB. Eosinophilic esophagitis in a patient with vigorous achalasia. Gastroenterology 1978;74:1298–301.
2. Mackenzie SH, Go M, Chadwick B, et al. Eosinophilic oesophagitis in patients presenting with dysphagia–a prospective analysis. Aliment Pharmacol Ther 2008;28:1140–6.
3. Prasad GA, Talley NJ, Romero Y, et al. Prevalence and predictive factors of eosinophilic esophagitis in patients presenting with dysphagia: a prospective study. Am J Gastroenterol 2007;102:2627–32.
4. Veerappan GR, Perry JL, Duncan TJ, et al. Prevalence of eosinophilic esophagitis in an adult population undergoing upper endoscopy: a prospective study. Clin Gastroenterol Hepatol 2009;7:420–6, 426.e1–2.
5. Croese J, Fairley SK, Masson JW, et al. Clinical and endoscopic features of eosinophilic esophagitis in adults. Gastrointest Endosc 2003;58:516–22.
6. Teriaky A, AlNasser A, McLean C, et al. The utility of endoscopic biopsies in patients with normal upper endoscopy. Can J Gastroenterol Hepatol 2016;2016: 3026563.
7. Dellon ES, Cotton CC, Gebhart JH, et al. Accuracy of the eosinophilic esophagitis endoscopic reference score in diagnosis and determining response to treatment. Clin Gastroenterol Hepatol 2016;14:31–9.
8. Savarino EV, Tolone S, Bartolo O, et al. The GerdQ questionnaire and high resolution manometry support the hypothesis that proton pump inhibitor-responsive oesophageal eosinophilia is a GERD-related phenomenon. Aliment Pharmacol Ther 2016;44:522–30.
9. Hirano I, Moy N, Heckman MG, et al. Endoscopic assessment of the oesophageal features of eosinophilic oesophagitis: validation of a novel classification and grading system. Gut 2013;62:489–95.

10. Kim HP, Vance RB, Shaheen NJ, et al. The prevalence and diagnostic utility of endoscopic features of eosinophilic esophagitis: a meta-analysis. Clin Gastroenterol Hepatol 2012;10:988–96.e5.
11. Schoepfer AM, Safroneeva E, Bussmann C, et al. Delay in diagnosis of eosinophilic esophagitis increases risk for stricture formation in a time-dependent manner. Gastroenterology 2013;145:1230–6.e2.
12. Gentile N, Katzka D, Ravi K, et al. Oesophageal narrowing is common and frequently under-appreciated at endoscopy in patients with oesophageal eosinophilia. Aliment Pharmacol Ther 2014;40:1333–40.
13. Kwiatek MA, Hirano I, Kahrilas PJ, et al. Mechanical properties of the esophagus in eosinophilic esophagitis. Gastroenterology 2011;140:82–90.
14. Kaplan M, Mutlu EA, Jakate S, et al. Endoscopy in eosinophilic esophagitis: "feline" esophagus and perforation risk. Clin Gastroenterol Hepatol 2003;1: 433–7.
15. Dellon ES, Gebhart JH, Higgins LL, et al. The esophageal biopsy "pull" sign: a highly specific and treatment-responsive endoscopic finding in eosinophilic esophagitis (with video). Gastrointest Endosc 2016;83:92–100.
16. Potter JW, Saeian K, Staff D, et al. Eosinophilic esophagitis in adults: an emerging problem with unique esophageal features. Gastrointest Endosc 2004;59:355–61.
17. Straumann A, Conus S, Degen L, et al. Budesonide is effective in adolescent and adult patients with active eosinophilic esophagitis. Gastroenterology 2010;139: 1526–37.
18. Dellon ES, Sheikh A, Speck O, et al. Viscous topical is more effective than nebulized steroid therapy for patients with eosinophilic esophagitis. Gastroenterology 2012;143:321–4.e1.
19. Alexander JA, Jung KW, Arora AS, et al. Swallowed fluticasone improves histologic but not symptomatic response of adults with eosinophilic esophagitis. Clin Gastroenterol Hepatol 2012;10:742–9.e1.
20. Francis DL, Foxx-Orenstein A, Arora AS, et al. Results of ambulatory pH monitoring do not reliably predict response to therapy in patients with eosinophilic oesophagitis. Aliment Pharmacol Ther 2012;35:300–7.
21. Moawad FJ, Veerappan GR, Dias JA, et al. Randomized controlled trial comparing aerosolized swallowed fluticasone to esomeprazole for esophageal eosinophilia. Am J Gastroenterol 2013;108:366–72.
22. Rodriguez-Sanchez J, Barrio-Andres J, Nantes Castillejo O, et al. The Endoscopic Reference Score shows modest accuracy to predict either clinical or histological activity in adult patients with eosinophilic oesophagitis. Aliment Pharmacol Ther 2017;45:300–9.
23. van Rhijn BD, Verheij J, Smout AJ, et al. The Endoscopic Reference Score shows modest accuracy to predict histologic remission in adult patients with eosinophilic esophagitis. Neurogastroenterol Motil 2016;28:1714–22.
24. Lee J, Huprich J, Kujath C, et al. Esophageal diameter is decreased in some patients with eosinophilic esophagitis and might increase with topical corticosteroid therapy. Clin Gastroenterol Hepatol 2012;10:481–6.
25. Carlson D, Hirano I, Zalewski A, et al. Changes in esophageal distensibility associated with treatment responds in eosinophilic esophagitis: a study utilizing the functional lumen imaging probe. Gastroenterology 2017;152(Supplement 1): S208.
26. Salek J, Clayton F, Vinson L, et al. Endoscopic appearance and location dictate diagnostic yield of biopsies in eosinophilic oesophagitis. Aliment Pharmacol Ther 2015;41:1288–95.

27. Straumann A, Spichtin HP, Grize L, et al. Natural history of primary eosinophilic esophagitis: a follow-up of 30 adult patients for up to 11.5 years. Gastroenterology 2003;125:1660–9.
28. Chehade M, Sampson HA, Morotti RA, et al. Esophageal subepithelial fibrosis in children with eosinophilic esophagitis. J Pediatr Gastroenterol Nutr 2007;45: 319–28.
29. Aceves SS, Newbury RO, Dohil R, et al. Esophageal remodeling in pediatric eosinophilic esophagitis. J Allergy Clin Immunol 2007;119:206–12.

# Eosinophilic Esophagitis in Children and Adults

Jonathan E. Markowitz, MD, MSCE[a],*, Steven B. Clayton, MD[b]

## KEYWORDS

- Eosinophilic esophagitis • Children • Adults • Clinical features • Treatment
- Diet therapy • Dilation

## KEY POINTS

- Adults and children with eosinophilic esophagitis (EoE) have distinct clinical and endoscopic presentations.
- Clinical presentation depends greatly on patient age.
- Treatments for EoE are effective across all age groups but used differently among pediatric and adult specialists.

## INTRODUCTION

Eosinophilic esophagitis (EoE) is a clinicohistologic diagnosis requiring both esophageal dysfunction and esophageal mucosal biopsies that demonstrate eosinophilia, without an alternative cause.[1] EoE is a prevalent cause of esophageal dysfunction in both children and adults.

Rarely described before 1993, EoE is the most prevalent eosinophilic gastrointestinal illness. It is the second major cause of esophagitis after gastroesophageal reflux disease (GERD) and EoE is the dominant cause of food impaction in young patients.[2] Initially, EoE was thought to be primarily a pediatric illness but later it was recognized in adults.

At first, esophageal eosinophilia was thought to be associated with reflux.[3–7] After the first multidisciplinary conference on EoE in Orlando, Florida, in 2005, EoE was recognized with increased frequency as a common cause of chronic dysphagia and esophageal symptoms in both children and adults.[7,8]

EoE affects all ages; clinical presentation depends greatly on the patient's ability to report symptoms associated with esophageal dysfunction. Recognition of clinical

[a] Pediatric Gastroenterology and Nutrition, Children's Hospital of Greenville Health System, University of South Carolina School of Medicine-Greenville, 200 Patewood Drive, Suite A-140, Greenville, SC 29615, USA; [b] Gastroenterology and Liver Center, Greenville Health System, University of South Carolina School of Medicine-Greenville, 890 West Faris Road, Suite 100, Greenville, SC 29605, USA
* Corresponding author.
E-mail address: JMarkowitz@ghs.org

Gastrointest Endoscopy Clin N Am 28 (2018) 59–75
http://dx.doi.org/10.1016/j.giec.2017.07.004
1052-5157/18/© 2017 Elsevier Inc. All rights reserved.

signs, along with laboratory and endoscopic findings, is critical for the identification of patients with EoE because delay in diagnosis has been associated with esophageal remodeling and stricture formation.[9–11]

This article describes the similarities and differences in clinical presentation of children and adults with EoE, including areas of epidemiology, clinical and endoscopic presentation, pathophysiology, and treatment.

## EPIDEMIOLOGIC ASPECTS OF EOSINOPHILIC ESOPHAGITIS

EoE was likely first described in the adult population as anecdotal cases of small-caliber esophagus found radiographically. However, the first identification of EoE as a separate and distinct disease entity began when Kelly and colleagues[12] identified a cohort of pediatric subjects with refractory esophagitis, characterized by eos, who failed to respond to acid suppression but went into remission when fed an elemental diet. From that point forward, esophagitis characterized by eosinophil (eos)-predominant inflammation has been studied extensively in both the pediatric and adult populations.

The first population-based studies of EoE in children were published in the early 2000s, with numerous additional cohort-based studies that have provided insight into the clinical features of patients with EoE, as well as population-based metrics. EoE has been described in people living in North America, South America, Europe, Asia, and Australia. EoE seems to be more prevalent among developed countries with higher socioeconomic development. However, within these countries, there is variation in prevalence rates, suggesting additional factors, such as climate, urban versus rural environment, and diet. An analysis of an esophageal biopsy database demonstrated a higher prevalence of EoE in cold climate zones of the United States.[13]

EoE has consistently demonstrated a strong male predominance in both adults and children, with a male to female ratio usually between 2.5:1 and 3:1. EoE has been diagnosed in every age group, ranging from infants to the elderly. In the pediatric population, the average age of diagnosis is typically between 6 and 10 years of age. Traditionally, there was a relatively long time lag before diagnosis (approximately 4 years), although this may be decreasing as awareness of the disease increases, not just among specialists who confirm the diagnosis but among primary care providers who make referrals.

Noel and colleagues[14] published the first population-based results on pediatric EoE in 2004. Evaluating a pathology database for histologic cases of isolated, esophageal eosinophilia (>24 eos per microscopic high-power field [HPF]), 315 cases of possible EoE were identified between 1991 and 2003. Almost all of those patients ($\sim$97%) were found after the year 2000, providing evidence that the disease was undergoing a significant increase in incidence. Further, in the 4-year period from 2000 to 2003, the incidence increased 4-fold (from 1 case to 4.3 cases per 10,000).

The largest detailed pediatric cohort with EoE was described in 2009 by Spergel and colleagues.[15] In this group of subjects followed at the Children's Hospital of Philadelphia, there was a steady increase in new diagnoses each year from 1996 to 2006. Excluding the patients referred from outside of their local area (PA, NJ, and DE) did not affect the pattern of newly diagnosed patients, suggesting referral bias was not a factor in the increase. The average age of diagnosis in this group was 6 years, with more than one-third of the patients younger than age 3 years at the time of diagnosis. Environmental allergies were thought to be a contributor to EoE findings in about 10% of the patients based on seasonal variation in biopsy findings without changes in diet or medical therapy.

Initially, EoE was considered predominantly a disease of children but, in 2008, a large national pathology database (Caris Diagnostics, Irving, TX, USA) was used to identify EoE cases. The study revealed that most EoE patients were 30 to 40 years old.[9] Current estimates of EoE prevalence vary widely in the literature. Dellon and colleagues[16] performed a large insurance database study. They estimated that EoE overall prevalence in the United States is approximately 57 per 100,000 persons. When separated by age, they found the prevalence in children and adults was 50.5 per 100,000, and 58.9 per 100,000, respectively. Patients with atopic symptoms tended to be diagnosed earlier and, although atopy is common in EoE, it is by no means universal.[17]

In both pediatric and adults patients, EoE predominantly affects white patients (about 80% of patients with EoE), but some studies suggest EoE prevalence may mirror the racial demographics of the surrounding area.[18–20]

## CLINICAL PRESENTATION

Clinical presentation varies considerably between adults and children. Differences in clinical presentation occur according to patient age and the patient's ability to communicate symptoms associated with esophageal dysfunction.[14,21] Thus, infants and younger children (who cannot report dysphagia) present with irritability, food aversion, failure to thrive, vomiting, regurgitation, and both chest and abdominal pain, similar to GERD.

In 2008, a large database study in the United States identified heartburn and abdominal pain or dyspepsia as the main reported symptoms in 38.1% and 31% of pediatric patients with EoE, respectively.[9] In children 11 years and older, EoE starts to present similarly to adults with symptomatic dysphagia and food impaction. Children with an atopic background or food-allergies present with more severe esophageal symptoms and food impaction.[22]

In adolescents and adults, the predominant symptoms are solid food dysphagia, heartburn, chest pain, and food bolus impaction. Dysphagia is present in most adult cases; however, food impaction is the symptom that most often leads to a diagnosis.[9,23] After the onset of symptoms of esophageal dysfunction, the median diagnostic delay of EoE was 4 to 6 years in both children and adults.[17,19]

Physical examination may reveal signs of atopic disease, such as wheezing on auscultation, eczematous skin findings, or stigmata of allergic rhinitis. Abdominal examination is typically benign and many patients will have a normal examination.

Endoscopic features of children and adults with EoE may differ significantly. Children will typically have endoscopic findings of primarily inflammatory features, such as edematous mucosa, loss of vascular markings, white exudates, and longitudinal furrows.[19] Features of fibrostenosis are more commonly seen in adults. These features are thought to be the result of esophageal remodeling and include fixed rings, narrow-caliber esophagus, dominant esophageal strictures, and fragile esophageal mucosa.[5] Many experts describe these 2 different endoscopic appearances as distinct phenotypes (inflammatory and fibrostenotic). However, these 2 subsets more likely represent different stages of disease progression.[17] Evidence for this is provided by reports from Schoepfer and colleagues,[24] who demonstrated an association between untreated EoE and the formation of esophageal strictures, and Dellon and colleagues,[17] who found the risk for a fibrostenotic phenotype seems to double for every 10-year increase in age.

Some retarded growth has been reported in younger patients but, overall, EoE does not seem to influence the final height of patients, does not shorten life expectancy, and has no association with an increased risk of developing malignancy.[2,25,26]

## COMPARISON OF ATOPIC FEATURES BETWEEN CHILDREN AND ADULTS WITH EOSINOPHILIC ESOPHAGITIS

Both children and adult patients with EoE frequently present with concomitant allergic diseases (eg, asthma, eczema, allergic rhinitis).[27] The prevalence of synchronous atopic ailments in EoE patients has been estimated as high as 80% in some studies.[28] In 2014, Vernon and colleagues[27] found the most common coexisting atopic condition with EoE in both children and adults was allergic rhinitis. Atopic dermatitis (17%) was the least common condition. They found children had a higher rates of asthma when compared with adults (P<.05).

A 2007 study from Australia suggested that, as age increases in children with EoE, inhalant allergen sensitization increases.[28,29] The exact immune-pathogenesis for EoE is not known. There is a high degree of atopy in both children and adults with EoE. These patients tend to be polysensitized to several environmental allergens and food allergens. Esophageal eosinophilia has been demonstrated after intranasal cockroach and dust mite delivery in mice, suggesting aeroallergen exposure plays an important role in the development of EoE; however, further study is needed.[30]

Vernon and colleagues[27] found that, in both children and adults, the most common aeroallergen sensitizations were to trees and dust mites. Children were more sensitive to dog and cat, whereas adults were more sensitive to grass. In both children and adults, the most common sensitizations to food allergens are to milk, soybean, wheat, eggs, and nuts; in adults, additional sensitizations to tomato, carrots, and onions were also common.[27,30,31]

## HISTOPATHOLOGICAL FEATURES

As detailed in the consensus documents, EoE is a clinicopathologic entity. This means that, although there are specific histopathologic criteria required to confirm a diagnosis, these must also exist in the correct clinical setting.[8,19] Namely, there must be symptoms of esophageal dysfunction, otherwise unexplainable, in addition to an isolated esophageal eosinophilia with a density that is at least 15 eos per microscopic HPF equivalent to 400× magnification. Although this would seem a straight-forward threshold, the microscopic HPF is not standardized because different microscopes have different field sizes. Few studies include the actual microscopic field size as part of their text.[32] Although small variation in the size of an HPF may not matter when eos counts far exceed or fall short of the 15 eos threshold, borderline cases may be over-reported or under-reported based on equipment.

EoE may affect the esophagus in a patchy manner. It was initially suggested that eos density was higher in the midesophagus than distal esophagus in patients with EoE (as opposed to patients with esophageal eosinophilia caused by reflux), but a large retrospective analysis in pediatric patients showed the distal esophagus to have a denser eosinophilic infiltrate than the midesophagus in patients with EoE.[33] The density of eosinophilia also correlated with the presence of dysphagia as a presenting symptom, rather than more general reflux symptoms. Significant differences in eosinophilic infiltrate density in proximal versus distal esophagus have not been consistently demonstrated in adults.[34] Because of the patchy nature of the disease, sampling error may occur with routine biopsies. The sensitivity for detecting EoE increases as the number of biopsies obtained increases and when multiple regions of the esophagus are sampled. In a cohort of 30 pediatric subjects with established EoE, a single esophageal biopsy had a sensitivity to detect EoE (based on a density of at least 15 eos/HPF) of 73%, increasing to 97% with 3 biopsy specimens and 100% with 6 specimens.[35]

In addition to eos density, there are other histologic features that characterize patients with EoE. Among these are basal zone hyperplasia, eos abscesses, eos surface layering, dilated intercellular space (DIS), surface epithelial alteration, dyskeratotic epithelial cells, and lamina propria fibrosis. The presence of these features, in particular basal zone hyperplasia and DIS, correlate well with disease activity, and have been shown to be responsive to treatment.[36]

## FIBROUS REMODELING OF THE ESOPHAGUS IN EOSINOPHILIC ESOPHAGITIS

EoE is a chronic relapsing condition in both children and adults. The likelihood of developing significant fibrosis increases with every 10-year increase in age.[17] Although fibrogenesis is part of normal repair of injured subepithelial cells, extensive subepithelial fibrosis in the esophagi of adult and pediatric patients with EoE often occurs. The cause of fibrogenesis in EoE patients is not completely known but studies suggest that secretory products of eos and mast cells, cytokines (eg, interleukin [IL]-13, IL-4, IL-5, eotaxin-3, and transforming growth factor [TGF]-β), epithelial cells, and stromal cells in the esophagus are involved in the process.[37,38]

Signals from epithelial cells and immune cells regulate fibrogenesis. Type 2 T helper cell cytokines overproduced in EoE have a significant influence in esophageal remodeling. Patients with EoE have increased expression of TGF-β1 in their esophagi; TGF-β1 activates fibroblasts. Cytokines IL-4, IL-13, and TGF-β regulate periostin, an extracellular matrix protein, and ligand for integrins by its effects on eos or by activating fibrogenic genes in the esophagus, leading to esophageal remodeling.[38] Therefore, prolonged exposure to an allergen stimulates this inflammatory cascade and leads to the development of fibrosis, esophageal strictures, and diffuse esophageal narrowing.[39]

## TREATMENT OF PEDIATRIC AND ADULT PATIENTS
### Initial Management

Similar in children and adults, initial management of the patient with EoE depends on several factors, including the severity of symptoms, medical resources available to the patient and providers, the experience and preference of the treating physician, and the motivation and financial resources of the patient and their family. Among the most commonly used treatments are steroids (both systemic and topical), dietary elimination (empirical or directed based on allergy testing), elemental diet, and esophageal dilation. In addition, proton pump inhibitor (PPI) therapy should be used as a concomitant therapy to confirm that disease is not PPI-responsive esophageal eosinophilia (PPI-REE), and to minimize secondary reflux symptoms due to an abnormally functioning esophagus. Each treatment choice has potential benefits and can be justified based on the available published experience. Likewise, each has its liabilities.

### Corticosteroids

Systemic corticosteroids have been previously shown to be effective in treating several allergic disorders associated with increased eos, including asthma, eczema, and eosinophilic gastroenteritis in both children and adults.[40–42] In patients with EoE, several reports have demonstrated a rapid and complete improvement in symptoms and histology when they are treated with oral steroids, such as prednisone and methylprednisolone.[33,43]

The advantages of systemic steroids include ease of administration, rapid onset of response, and very high response rate. However, the toxicities relating to prolonged steroid use are well documented, and the high relapse rate of EoE after treatment is discontinued limit the utility of oral steroids as a maintenance therapy. Presently, systemic steroids should be reserved for isolated cases, such as patients who have esophageal strictures or small-caliber esophagus causing significant dysphagia, food impaction, weight loss, or severe swallowing problems that require a rapid treatment response before other treatments are instituted.

Topical corticosteroids were first suggested as a potential treatment of EoE a few years after systemic steroids were demonstrated to be effective.[44] The first trials of topical steroids used aerosolized forms of steroids originally developed for inhalation as a treatment of asthma. These aerosolized preparations were swallowed rather than inhaled, in an effort to coat the surface of the esophagus and limit systemic exposure. Utilization of budesonide in some preparations further reduced the likelihood of systemic side effects, owing to rapid first-pass hepatic metabolism.[45,46] Recent data suggest that viscous budesonide may offer advantages in terms of dose delivered directly to the esophagus (as opposed to ending up in the lungs), which may in turn lead to better anti-inflammatory activity.[47] The use of topical steroids proved to be successful in reducing symptoms, as well as eosinophilic inflammation.[48] However, as seen with systemic steroid therapy, the long-term success of topical steroids has been shown to be limited because symptoms and esophageal eosinophilia almost always recur when the medication is weaned or discontinued. Although significant side effects of topical steroids have yet to be reported, esophageal candidiasis has been seen in a proportion of patients who receive this therapy.[49] In addition, there are growing concerns about effects on growth in pediatric patients, as well as suppression of the hypothalamic-pituitary-adrenal axis.[50]

Because of the currently reported minimal risk of systemic side effects, many experts advocate ongoing treatment with topical steroids, whereas others suggest intermittent treatment. To date, there is no maintenance method that has been proven to be most effective. It also remains to be seen whether this therapeutic approach reduces esophageal inflammation enough to prevent long-term complications, such as fibrotic changes in the esophagus.

At this point, it seems that effectiveness of both forms of topical steroid therapy is comparable enough that selection should depend on a discussion between the physician, the patient, and his or her family.

### Dietary Therapy

From the time that EoE was first recognized, it was strongly suggested that it was an allergic disease. The original case series that demonstrated improvement in esophagitis on an elemental diet laid the groundwork for using restriction of food antigens as a treatment of EoE.[12] In that series, patients not only responded to an elemental diet but also developed a recurrence of symptoms when they were re-exposed to the offending foods. Subsequent studies have confirmed that restriction of food antigens can result in both a significant symptomatic and histologic improvement of EoE. Although there is little debate on these points, the difficulty lies in how best to determine which and how many food antigens are causing the clinical symptoms and esophageal eosinophilia.

### Elemental Diet

Among all of the methods for restricting foods from the diet, the administration of an elemental diet using a strict amino acid-based formula has shown the highest response rate both clinically and histologically in children. Multiple reports have demonstrated that greater than 95% of pediatric patients respond both clinically and histologically to the introduction of an elemental diet.[33,51] Reports suggest that symptom resolution may occur as quickly as within the first week of starting the diet. Follow-up biopsies,

1 month after starting treatment, show essentially complete resolution of eosinophilia in many cases. Of the commonly accepted treatments for EoE, treatment with elemental diet can be considered the most efficacious. However, the effectiveness of the diet, meaning the utility in real-world situations rather than controlled trials, may be limited because of several logistical issues associated with this treatment.

The greatest limitation to the use of an elemental diet is palatability. In general, the more elemental the protein source in a formula, the more unpalatable it tends to be. Further adding to the poor taste is the presence of a high proportion of medium-chain triglyceride oil and lack of sweet-tasting sugars. The initial versions of elemental formulas had a very strong taste and smell. When introduced early in life, children commonly adjust to the taste of elemental formulas; however, the initiation of these formulas in a child or adolescent who is already used to a more normal diet can be a difficult proposition. Newer generations of elemental formulas have eased this difficulty, to a degree, with much better palatability and a variety of flavors. Nevertheless, a strictly elemental formula diet is a difficult long-term approach. At 30 kcal/oz, the elemental formulas designed for use in children older than 1 year of age require relatively large volumes over the course of a day to provide adequate nutrition. A minimum of 1 L of formula is commonly administered in the smallest of children, whereas older children and adolescents may need 2 L or more of formula per day. In many cases, children are unable to drink this volume of formula, necessitating enteral tube feeding via nasogastric tubes, or a surgically or endoscopically placed gastrostomy tube.

Another problem is that the cost of elemental formulas tends to be higher than intact protein formulas or hydrolyzed protein formulas. The cost takes on more importance because insurance coverage for elemental diet in EoE varies from state to state, and plan to plan, leaving some families responsible for the full cost of the formulas. Although elemental diet is costly, these costs must be balanced with the long-term costs of medical therapy and evaluated over the long-term. Over time, dietary therapy tends to be less expensive than medical therapy.[52]

Emotional costs also exist because of quality-of-life issues. Using a strict elemental diet not only removes individuals from the social aspects of eating but also affects the rest of the family who may be asked to alter their diet in support of the patient. It is important that those who attempt to use an elemental diet receive close observation to ensure that their nutritional needs are being met. This includes total calories, as well as macronutrients and micronutrients. Nutritional deficiencies have been recognized in children on exclusive elemental diets for prolonged periods.[53] It is advisable that a pediatric dietitian or nutritionist, or a physician with expertise in nutritional management, oversee the administration of elemental diet to minimize the risks of this form of treatment. These patients may also need the support of social work, case management, psychology, and feeding specialists.

There are limited data on the effectiveness of elemental diet in adults with EoE; however, preliminary studies demonstrated improvement in symptoms, endoscopic appearance, and histologic response rates similar to pediatric trials. There were higher patient dropout rates due to unpalatability of the formula diet and nonadherence to the diet protocol.[54–56] Patient willingness to try the treatment and long-term adherence to the program are the biggest limiting factors, as opposed to efficacy, of elemental diet in the treatment of adults with EoE.

### Dietary Restriction

Despite the high success rate of elemental diets in EoE, there are numerous advantages to being able to eat an intact protein diet. Choosing which foods to restrict from the diet can be difficult, yet choosing correctly is vital to the success of this approach. The decision on how to restrict the diet also depends on the resources available to the patient. The 2 most common approaches to dietary restriction are an empirical diet (based on the removal of the most common problematic food antigens) and a directed diet (based on the results of allergy testing).

Empirical food elimination of the most common causative foods has been shown to be an effective approach in children. In 2006, Kagalwalla and colleagues[57] compared the clinical and histologic response of a 6-food elimination diet (SFED) that restricted cow's milk, soy protein, peanut or tree-nuts, wheat, eggs, and fish or shellfish to another cohort of EoE subjects who received an elemental diet. Of the SFED group, 74% showed a histologic response after a minimum of 6 weeks of treatment, with peak eos count dropping from about 80 eos per HPF to 13. Although these results were favorable, those who received an elemental diet over that time showed a more complete histologic response. Very similar results have been seen in adults administered the same diet, further suggesting that pediatric and adult EoE are similarly responsive to diet elimination.[31]

Meanwhile, directed dietary therapy has also been shown to be successful. Often, patients with EoE have reactions to multiple foods. Spergel and colleagues[58] demonstrated that many patients with EoE manifest evidence of both immediate-type (immunoglobulin [Ig]-E–mediated) and delayed-type (T-cell mediated) allergy. Traditional skin prick testing provides evidence of IgE-mediated food allergy, whereas atopy patch testing may provide supplemental data on delayed-type hypersensitivity reactions to foods. When used together, the sensitivity of these forms of testing tend to be high but the specificity is variable.

These tests increase the likelihood that specific dietary elimination will be successful; however, false positives and false negatives frequently occur. When used, the elimination of foods identified by testing is usually applied for a minimum of 4 to 6 weeks, followed by esophagogastroduodenoscopy (EGD) to confirm a histologic response. Although clinical improvement may take place within the first few weeks of food elimination, it remains critical to re-evaluate the mucosal response with biopsy in both clinical responders and nonresponders. It is not uncommon for symptoms to wax and wane even when inflammatory activity remains constant. Furthermore, because many symptoms of EoE are not specific to this disorder, it is important to confirm that ongoing symptoms are truly due to ongoing eosinophilic inflammation and not another cause, such as acid reflux.

As with elemental diet, it is highly advisable to have a dietitian available to the family that undertakes any dietary therapy, whether directed by allergy testing or empirical therapy. Just like the use of elemental formulas, restrictive diets put patients at risk for macronutrient and micronutrient deficiencies.[59] Additionally, the ubiquitous nature of certain types of food antigens, such as wheat, soy, and cow's milk, make complete elimination extremely difficult. A skilled dietitian who has experience counseling patients and their families on recognizing food antigens in ingredient lists can greatly help to prevent inadequate response due to inadvertent exposure to foods. Further support for patients can be provided through organizations such as the Food Allergy and Anaphylaxis Network (FAAN) and the American Partnership for Eosinophilic Disorders (APFED).

## SUGGESTED APPROACH TO PATIENTS WITH EOSINOPHILIC ESOPHAGITIS: CHILDREN VERSUS ADULTS

Adults and children with EoE have a distinct clinical and endoscopic presentation and, therefore, treatment varies between the 2 cohorts (**Table 1**). In both children and adults, the treatment of EoE pursues several endpoints:

**Table 1**
**Characteristics of eosinophilic esophagitis in children and adults**

|  | Children | Adults |
|---|---|---|
| Presenting symptoms | Failure to thrive<br>Feeding refusal<br>Regurgitation<br>Vomiting<br>Heartburn<br>Dysphagia<br>Food impaction | Heartburn<br>Dysphagia<br>Food impaction |
| Warning symptoms (to prompt early endoscopy) | Weight loss<br>Food impaction | Dysphagia<br>Food impaction |
| Proportion of patients with PPI-REE | Low | High |
| Most common endoscopic findings | Edema<br>Furrowing<br>White exudates | Rings<br>Stricture<br>Small-caliber esophagus |
| Most common treatments | Diet restriction<br>Elemental diet<br>Topical steroids | Topical steroids<br>Esophageal dilation |

1. Improvement of dysphagia and frequency of food bolus impactions
2. Histologic remission of the esophageal mucosal eosinophilia
3. Restoration of functional esophageal lumen diameter
4. Prevention of fibrosis and esophageal remodeling.[5,60]

## PEDIATRIC PATIENTS

Although there are differences in EoE among adult and pediatric patients relating to epidemiology, presentation, and other historical features, the main difference in the adult and pediatric populations relates to the way that the disease presents and is treated in the different age groups. These differences arise for several reasons but do not relate primarily to differential response to treatments between the adult and pediatric groups.

The lack of a consistent and sequential treatment strategy stems not only from a lack of head-to-head trials of treatments but also relates to differences such as whether the treating physician is a gastroenterologist or an allergist, the philosophy of the treating physician, the willingness of the patient to participate in specific treatment strategies, and the resources available to the patient and the treatment team. Understanding that there is no single accepted treatment approach, and that all treatments discussed have a reasonable expectation of success, the authors propose the following approaches to treating children and adults with EoE.

EGD with biopsy is the only standard with which the diagnosis of EoE can be made. Wherever possible in pediatric patients, EGD should be delayed until an adequate trial of acid suppression can be given to see if the symptoms of esophageal dysfunction resolve. A minimum of 4 weeks of therapy with a PPI given at high dose is preferred, with an 8-week trial considered optimal. In children, many experts in EoE suggest using twice daily dosing of a PPI, at a dose up to 1 mg/kg/dose, to a maximal adult dose. In circumstances in which the EGD is performed before an adequate trial of acid blockade, a subsequent trial of acid blockade and re-evaluation of the esophageal mucosa is considered necessary to confirm the non-PPI responsive form of esophageal eosinophilia.

Following a diagnosis of EoE in children, either dietary restriction or elimination, or the use of topical steroids, should be instituted. In certain circumstances, such as a significant small-caliber esophagus or multiple food impactions, a more aggressive initial treatment approach, such as systemic steroids or esophageal dilatation, may be needed.

Often, the therapeutic choice is made depending on the resources of the physician and after a discussion with the patient and family. When considering the use of diet restriction or elimination, in cases in which allergy testing does not reveal any potential foods for removal or cases in which the dietary restrictions prove too difficult for the family to maintain, topical steroid therapy should be considered. Alternatively, in patients who are unable to comply with using topical steroids, dietary restrictions should be considered. During any therapy, a repeat EGD is recommended (minimum 4–8 weeks later) to document resolution of inflammation. As previously mentioned, close follow-up is required regardless of treatment choice. When using dietary restrictions, one must make sure that adequate nutrition is supplied and that growth is maintained.

When using steroids, medication side effects and growth also require monitoring. After the initiation of therapy, the authors advise that acid suppression be maintained throughout the treatment process until a final course of therapy has been chosen. With regard to topical steroid therapy, initial dosing is usually twice daily. The duration of treatment with topical steroids remains unclear but it is widely believed that disease almost always relapses on discontinuation of treatment. Most EoE experts advocate decreasing the dosing schedule once symptoms are controlled and inflammation improves. Topical steroid therapy should be maintained as long as is necessary to maintain a symptomatic remission. Some clinicians will choose to discontinue therapy periodically, with a plan to restart treatment once symptoms re-emerge.

A repeat EGD is recommended after medication changes (minimum 4–8 weeks) to document resolution of inflammation. Presently, it remains unclear what degree of eosinophilia presents a risk for long-term complications, such as esophageal fibrosis and stricture formation, but it is generally thought that lower numbers of eos are better.

With regard to dietary elimination, once remission is achieved with dietary therapy, food challenges with restricted foods can be started. Symptom relapse following introduction of a previously restricted food is adequate to define failure on reintroduction, but lack of symptoms does not ensure that disease has not relapsed. After the introduction of a single or a small group of foods, an endoscopy should be performed to confirm that there has not been a subclinical relapse. The number of foods to be introduced before endoscopy is a matter of choice. Endoscopy between each food introduction is the most definitive way to evaluate each food, but is costly and results in cumulatively greater, albeit low, procedural risk (including additional anesthesia). However, the more foods introduced between each endoscopy introduce less certainty as to which food or foods are responsible if a relapse is found. As a guideline, it is reasonable to introduce a few lower-risk foods at a time between endoscopy, while performing endoscopy between introductions of higher risk single foods or foods that are more of a staple of the typical diet, such as egg, milk, and wheat.

## ADULT PATIENTS

In adult patients, dysphagia is considered an alarm symptom and warrants an EGD to evaluate for underlying malignancy that could be causing an anatomic esophageal obstruction.[61] Adults with EoE tend to present with dysphagia and food bolus impaction and, therefore, adults typically will undergo endoscopy before a 2-month trial of

PPIs. In adult patients with endoscopic features of EoE, it is recommended that esophageal biopsies should be targeted to areas of endoscopic abnormality, mainly white exudates and longitudinal furrows, which are associated with higher peak eos counts. At least 6 biopsies should be obtained from at least 2 different locations in the esophagus.[62] From 2006 to 2010, several retrospective case series and studies highlighted the existence of patients with clinical, endoscopic, and histologic features compatible with EoE showing clinicopathological response to PPI therapy. Similar findings have been reported in children.[62] Therefore, consensus guidelines recommend evaluating for PPI-REE. PPI-REE is considered when patients have esophageal symptoms and have histologic findings of esophageal eosinophilia but demonstrate symptomatic and histologic response to proton pump inhibition. To exclude PPI-REE, patients with esophageal eosinophilia should be given a 2-month course of PPIs followed by endoscopy with repeat biopsy to assess for resolution or persistence of esophageal eosinophilia. If there is persistent eosinophilia and symptoms of esophageal dysfunction, then EoE can be formally diagnosed.[1,62]

The treatment of the inflammatory component in EoE serves to document histologic remission of the esophageal mucosal eosinophilia and prevent development of fibrosis and esophageal remodeling, and is similar in both adult and pediatric patients. Diet elimination and swallowed corticosteroids are used in a similar fashion in both groups with the goal of symptom and esophageal mucosal eosinophilia resolution. This section focuses on key areas of differences in treatment between the 2 groups. **Fig. 1** is a suggested algorithm for diagnosis and treatment of EoE in adults.

Given the higher prevalence of the fibrostenotic subtype in adults compared with children, this is where the treatment of EoE varies between the pediatric population and adults the most.[19,63] EoE is thought to be a chronic progressive disease.[11,26,64,65] After symptom onset, patients present initially with an inflammatory phenotype with a normal esophageal lumen diameter. However, without treatment, the fibrostenotic phenotype prevalence exceeds 82% after 10 to 15 years of disease onset and 100% after 15-year delay.[11] Dysphagia from EoE in adults is usually multifactorial and is secondary to esophageal mucosal inflammation, fibrostenotic esophageal remodeling, and some degree of esophageal dysmotility.[5,66,67] Therefore, in adults, a single treatment type rarely adequately treats all the facets of the disease and multiple treatment modalities are often used, especially in patients with the fibrostenotic phenotype.[5,68]

The key features of the fibrostenotic subtype of EoE are narrow-caliber esophagus, esophageal rings, and focal esophageal strictures.[69] The reduction in the esophageal lumen diameter increases resistance to bolus transit along the length of the esophagus. According to the Poiseuille law ($R = 8 \, \eta^* L / r^{\wedge}4$) esophageal outflow resistance (R) is directly proportional to the length (L) of the esophagus and the viscosity ($\eta$) of the bolus, and inversely proportional to the radius to the fourth power. Therefore, there are 3 primary factors that determine the resistance to bolus transit within the esophagus: esophageal diameter (or radius), esophageal length, and viscosity of the bolus.

Of these 3 factors, the most important quantitatively and physiologically is esophageal diameter. A change in esophageal luminal diameter exponentially alters resistance. Therefore, subtle changes in esophageal lumen diameter result in significant elevation in resistance to bolus transit in EoE patients.[66] Restoring the functional esophageal lumen diameter is of key importance when treating adults with the fibrostenotic subtype.

Esophageal dilation is an effective treatment of esophageal narrowing in adult patients with the fibrostenotic subtype of EoE.[1,19,68] Earlier reports on performing dilation in subjects with EoE described a higher than expected rate of

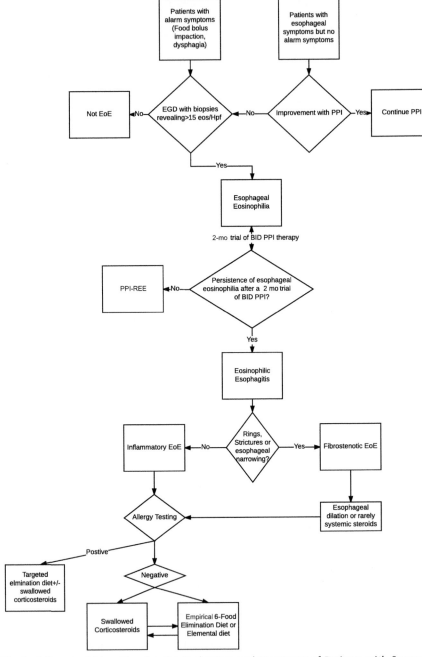

**Fig. 1.** A Proposed Algorithm for the Evaluation and Treatment of Patients with Suspected Eosinophilic Esophagitis.

complications.[70,71] In 2017, a large meta-analysis of 27 studies demonstrated that endoscopic dilation is consistently effective in children and adults with EoE, resulting in symptom improvement in 95% of subjects with very low rates (<1%) of major complications.[68]

Few data exist to support a single specific method of esophageal dilation over another.[1] The authors recommend bougie dilation because of the ability to dilate multiple strictures and long strictures, as seen in a diffusely narrowed esophagus in EoE. The goal of dilation therapy is to start with a small diameter bougie or balloon, progress slowly, and gradually dilate to a diameter of 15 to 18 mm to achieve symptom relief.[5] Common and expected adverse effects after dilation in EoE are mucosal tears and chest pain. These occur because the goal of dilation therapy is to disrupt fibrotic esophageal remodeling and increase the functional lumen diameter of the esophagus.[72] After reaching an optimal esophageal lumen diameter, repeat endoscopic dilatations should be considered after symptoms begin to recur.

## SUMMARY

Adults and children with EoE have distinct clinical and endoscopic presentations. Recognition of clinical signs, along with laboratory and endoscopic findings, is critical for the identification of patients with EoE because delay in diagnosis has been associated with esophageal remodeling and stricture formation. Clinical presentation varies considerably between adults and children but more due to differences in the patients than to differences in the disease. Clinical presentation changes according to patient's age and the patient's ability to communicate symptoms associated with esophageal dysfunction. The higher prevalence of the fibrostenotic subtype in adults compared with children likely relates more to duration of disease than to different phenotypes. The need for dilation therapy to disrupt fibrotic esophageal remodeling and increase the functional lumen diameter of the esophagus is a major difference in treatment between the 2 groups. However, early and accurate diagnosis, in combination with effective treatment can lead to symptom and disease remission in both children and adults with EoE.

## REFERENCES

1. Dellon ES, Gonsalves N, Hirano I, et al. ACG clinical guideline: Evidenced based approach to the diagnosis and management of esophageal eosinophilia and eosinophilic esophagitis (EoE). Am J Gastroenterol 2013;108(5):679–92 [quiz: 693].
2. Lucendo AJ, Sanchez-Cazalilla M. Adult versus pediatric eosinophilic esophagitis: important differences and similarities for the clinician to understand. Expert Rev Clin Immunol 2012;8(8):733–45.
3. Liacouras CA. Eosinophilic esophagitis in children and adults. J Pediatr Gastroenterol Nutr 2003;37(Suppl 1):S23–8.
4. Landres RT, Kuster GG, Strum WB. Eosinophilic esophagitis in a patient with vigorous achalasia. Gastroenterology 1978;74(6):1298–301.
5. Richter JE. Current management of eosinophilic esophagitis 2015. J Clin Gastroenterol 2016;50(2):99–110.
6. Winter HS, Madara JL, Stafford RJ, et al. Intraepithelial eosinophils: a new diagnostic criterion for reflux esophagitis. Gastroenterology 1982;83(4):818–23.
7. Attwood SE, Smyrk TC, Demeester TR, et al. Esophageal eosinophilia with dysphagia. A distinct clinicopathologic syndrome. Dig Dis Sci 1993;38(1):109–16.

8. Furuta GT, Liacouras CA, Collins MH, et al. Eosinophilic esophagitis in children and adults: a systematic review and consensus recommendations for diagnosis and treatment. Gastroenterology 2007;133(4):1342–63.

9. Kapel RC, Miller JK, Torres C, et al. Eosinophilic esophagitis: a prevalent disease in the United States that affects all age groups. Gastroenterology 2008;134(5): 1316–21.

10. Putnam PE. Eosinophilic esophagitis in children: clinical manifestations. Gastrointest Endosc Clin N Am 2008;18(1):11–23, vii.

11. Lipka S, Kumar A, Richter JE. Impact of diagnostic delay and other risk factors on eosinophilic esophagitis phenotype and esophageal diameter. J Clin Gastroenterol 2016;50(2):134–40.

12. Kelly KJ, Lazenby AJ, Rowe PC, et al. Eosinophilic esophagitis attributed to gastroesophageal reflux: improvement with an amino acid-based formula. Gastroenterology 1995;109(5):1503–12.

13. Hurrell JM, Genta RM, Dellon ES. Prevalence of esophageal eosinophilia varies by climate zone in the United States. Am J Gastroenterol 2012;107(5):698–706.

14. Noel RJ, Putnam PE, Rothenberg ME. Eosinophilic esophagitis. N Engl J Med 2004;351(9):940–1.

15. Spergel JM, Brown-Whitehorn TF, Beausoleil JL, et al. 14 years of eosinophilic esophagitis: clinical features and prognosis. J Pediatr Gastroenterol Nutr 2009; 48(1):30–6.

16. Dellon ES, Jensen ET, Martin CF, et al. Prevalence of eosinophilic esophagitis in the United States. Clin Gastroenterol Hepatol 2014;12(4):589–96.e1.

17. Dellon ES, Kim HP, Sperry SL, et al. A phenotypic analysis shows that eosinophilic esophagitis is a progressive fibrostenotic disease. Gastrointest Endosc 2014; 79(4):577–85.e4.

18. Sperry SL, Woosley JT, Shaheen NJ, et al. Influence of race and gender on the presentation of eosinophilic esophagitis. Am J Gastroenterol 2012;107(2): 215–21.

19. Liacouras CA, Furuta GT, Hirano I, et al. Eosinophilic esophagitis: updated consensus recommendations for children and adults. J Allergy Clin Immunol 2011;128(1):3–20.e6 [quiz: 21–2].

20. Hruz P. Epidemiology of eosinophilic esophagitis. Dig Dis 2014;32(1–2):40–7.

21. Putnam PE. Eosinophilic esophagitis in children: clinical manifestations. Gastroenterol Clin North Am 2008;37(2):369–81, vi.

22. DeBrosse CW, Franciosi JP, King EC, et al. Long-term outcomes in pediatric-onset esophageal eosinophilia. J Allergy Clin Immunol 2011;128(1):132–8.

23. Katzka DA. Demographic data and symptoms of eosinophilic esophagitis in adults. Gastrointest Endosc Clin N Am 2008;18(1):25–32, viii.

24. Schoepfer AM, Safroneeva E, Bussmann C, et al. Delay in diagnosis of eosinophilic esophagitis increases risk for stricture formation in a time-dependent manner. Gastroenterology 2013;145(6):1230–6.e1-2.

25. Squires KA, Cameron DJ, Oliver M, et al. Herpes simplex and eosinophilic oesophagitis: the chicken or the egg? J Pediatr Gastroenterol Nutr 2009;49(2):246–50.

26. Straumann A, Spichtin HP, Grize L, et al. Natural history of primary eosinophilic esophagitis: a follow-up of 30 adult patients for up to 11.5 years. Gastroenterology 2003;125(6):1660–9.

27. Vernon N, Shah S, Lehman E, et al. Comparison of atopic features between children and adults with eosinophilic esophagitis. Allergy Asthma Proc 2014;35(5): 409–14.

28. Sugnanam KK, Collins JT, Smith PK, et al. Dichotomy of food and inhalant allergen sensitization in eosinophilic esophagitis. Allergy 2007;62(11):1257–60.
29. Erwin EA, James HR, Gutekunst HM, et al. Serum IgE measurement and detection of food allergy in pediatric patients with eosinophilic esophagitis. Ann Allergy Asthma Immunol 2010;104(6):496–502.
30. Roy-Ghanta S, Larosa DF, Katzka DA. Atopic characteristics of adult patients with eosinophilic esophagitis. Clin Gastroenterol Hepatol 2008;6(5):531–5.
31. Gonsalves N, Yang GY, Doerfler B, et al. Elimination diet effectively treats eosinophilic esophagitis in adults; food reintroduction identifies causative factors. Gastroenterology 2012;142(7):1451–9.e1 [quiz: e14–5].
32. Sperry SL, Shaheen NJ, Dellon ES. Toward uniformity in the diagnosis of eosinophilic esophagitis (EoE): the effect of guidelines on variability of diagnostic criteria for EoE. Am J Gastroenterol 2011;106(5):824–32 [quiz: 833].
33. Liacouras CA, Spergel JM, Ruchelli E, et al. Eosinophilic esophagitis: a 10-year experience in 381 children. Clin Gastroenterol Hepatol 2005;3(12):1198–206.
34. Lucendo AJ, Arias A, De Rezende LC, et al. Subepithelial collagen deposition, profibrogenic cytokine gene expression, and changes after prolonged fluticasone propionate treatment in adult eosinophilic esophagitis: a prospective study. J Allergy Clin Immunol 2011;128(5):1037–46.
35. Shah A, Kagalwalla AF, Gonsalves N, et al. Histopathologic variability in children with eosinophilic esophagitis. Am J Gastroenterol 2009;104(3):716–21.
36. Collins MH, Martin LJ, Alexander ES, et al. Newly developed and validated eosinophilic esophagitis histology scoring system and evidence that it outperforms peak eosinophil count for disease diagnosis and monitoring. Dis Esophagus 2017;30(3):1–8.
37. Chehade M, Sampson HA, Morotti RA, et al. Esophageal subepithelial fibrosis in children with eosinophilic esophagitis. J Pediatr Gastroenterol Nutr 2007;45(3):319–28.
38. Cheng E, Souza RF, Spechler SJ. Tissue remodeling in eosinophilic esophagitis. Am J Physiol Gastrointest Liver Physiol 2012;303(11):G1175–87.
39. Hill DA, Spergel JM. The immunologic mechanisms of eosinophilic esophagitis. Curr Allergy Asthma Rep 2016;16(2):9.
40. Markowitz JE, Russo P, Liacouras CA. Solitary duodenal ulcer: a new presentation of eosinophilic gastroenteritis. Gastrointest Endosc 2000;52(5):673–6.
41. Park HS, Kim HS, Jang HJ. Eosinophilic gastroenteritis associated with food allergy and bronchial asthma. J Korean Med Sci 1995;10(3):216–9.
42. Redondo-Cerezo E, Cabello MJ, Gonzalez Y, et al. Eosinophilic gastroenteritis: our recent experience: one-year experience of atypical onset of an uncommon disease. Scand J Gastroenterol 2001;36(12):1358–60.
43. Liacouras CA, Wenner WJ, Brown K, et al. Primary eosinophilic esophagitis in children: successful treatment with oral corticosteroids. J Pediatr Gastroenterol Nutr 1998;26(4):380–5.
44. Faubion WA Jr, Perrault J, Burgart LJ, et al. Treatment of eosinophilic esophagitis with inhaled corticosteroids. J Pediatr Gastroenterol Nutr 1998;27(1):90–3.
45. Aceves SS, Bastian JF, Newbury RO, et al. Oral viscous budesonide: a potential new therapy for eosinophilic esophagitis in children. Am J Gastroenterol 2007;102(10):2271–9 [quiz: 2280].
46. Aceves SS, Dohil R, Newbury RO, et al. Topical viscous budesonide suspension for treatment of eosinophilic esophagitis. J Allergy Clin Immunol 2005;116(3):705–6.

47. Dellon ES, Sheikh A, Speck O, et al. Viscous topical is more effective than nebulized steroid therapy for patients with eosinophilic esophagitis. Gastroenterology 2012;143(2):321–4.e1.
48. Dohil R, Newbury R, Fox L, et al. Oral viscous budesonide is effective in children with eosinophilic esophagitis in a randomized, placebo-controlled trial. Gastroenterology 2010;139(2):418–29.
49. Teitelbaum JE, Fox VL, Twarog FJ, et al. Eosinophilic esophagitis in children: immunopathological analysis and response to fluticasone propionate. Gastroenterology 2002;122(5):1216–25.
50. Ahmet A, Benchimol EI, Goldbloom EB, et al. Adrenal suppression in children treated with swallowed fluticasone and oral viscous budesonide for eosinophilic esophagitis. Allergy Asthma Clin Immunol 2016;12:49.
51. Markowitz JE, Spergel JM, Ruchelli E, et al. Elemental diet is an effective treatment for eosinophilic esophagitis in children and adolescents. Am J Gastroenterol 2003;98(4):777–82.
52. Cotton CC, Erim D, Eluri S, et al. Cost utility analysis of topical steroids compared with dietary elimination for treatment of eosinophilic esophagitis. Clin Gastroenterol Hepatol 2017;15(6):841–9.e1.
53. Jones M, Campbell KA, Duggan C, et al. Multiple micronutrient deficiencies in a child fed an elemental formula. J Pediatr Gastroenterol Nutr 2001;33(5):602–5.
54. Kavitt RT, Hirano I, Vaezi MF. Diagnosis and treatment of eosinophilic esophagitis in adults. Am J Med 2016;129(9):924–34.
55. Molina-Infante J, Martin-Noguerol E, Alvarado-Arenas M, et al. Selective elimination diet based on skin testing has suboptimal efficacy for adult eosinophilic esophagitis. J Allergy Clin Immunol 2012;130(5):1200–2.
56. Peterson KA, Byrne KR, Vinson LA, et al. Elemental diet induces histologic response in adult eosinophilic esophagitis. Am J Gastroenterol 2013;108(5):759–66.
57. Kagalwalla AF, Sentongo TA, Ritz S, et al. Effect of six-food elimination diet on clinical and histologic outcomes in eosinophilic esophagitis. Clin Gastroenterol Hepatol 2006;4(9):1097–102.
58. Spergel JM, Andrews T, Brown-Whitehorn TF, et al. Treatment of eosinophilic esophagitis with specific food elimination diet directed by a combination of skin prick and patch tests. Ann Allergy Asthma Immunol 2005;95(4):336–43.
59. Noimark L, Cox HE. Nutritional problems related to food allergy in childhood. Pediatr Allergy Immunol 2008;19(2):188–95.
60. Prieto R, Richter JE. Eosinophilic esophagitis in adults: an update on medical management. Curr Gastroenterol Rep 2013;15(6):324.
61. Fransen GA, Janssen MJ, Muris JW, et al. Meta-analysis: the diagnostic value of alarm symptoms for upper gastrointestinal malignancy. Aliment Pharmacol Ther 2004;20(10):1045–52.
62. Lucendo AJ, Molina-Infante J, Arias A, et al. Guidelines on eosinophilic esophagitis: evidence-based statements and recommendations for diagnosis and management in children and adults. United European Gastroenterol J 2017;5(3):335–58.
63. Gonsalves N. Distinct features in the clinical presentations of eosinophilic esophagitis in children and adults: is this the same disease? Dig Dis 2014;32(1–2):89–92.
64. Aceves SS, Newbury RO, Dohil R, et al. Esophageal remodeling in pediatric eosinophilic esophagitis. J Allergy Clin Immunol 2007;119(1):206–12.

65. Mishra A, Wang M, Pemmaraju VR, et al. Esophageal remodeling develops as a consequence of tissue specific IL-5-induced eosinophilia. Gastroenterology 2008;134(1):204–14.
66. Colizzo JM, Clayton SB, Richter JE. Intrabolus pressure on high-resolution manometry distinguishes fibrostenotic and inflammatory phenotypes of eosinophilic esophagitis. Dis Esophagus 2016;29(6):551–7.
67. von Arnim U, Kandulski A, Weigt J, et al. Correlation of high-resolution manometric findings with symptoms of dysphagia and endoscopic features in adults with eosinophilic esophagitis. Dig Dis 2017;35(5):472–7.
68. Moawad FJ, Molina-Infante J, Lucendo AJ, et al. Systematic review with meta-analysis: endoscopic dilation is highly effective and safe in children and adults with eosinophilic oesophagitis. Aliment Pharmacol Ther 2017;46(2):96–105.
69. Hirano I, Moy N, Heckman MG, et al. Endoscopic assessment of the oesophageal features of eosinophilic oesophagitis: validation of a novel classification and grading system. Gut 2013;62(4):489–95.
70. Kaplan M, Mutlu EA, Jakate S, et al. Endoscopy in eosinophilic esophagitis: "feline" esophagus and perforation risk. Clin Gastroenterol Hepatol 2003;1(6):433–7.
71. Lucendo AJ, De Rezende L. Endoscopic dilation in eosinophilic esophagitis: a treatment strategy associated with a high risk of perforation. Endoscopy 2007;39(4):376 [author reply: 377].
72. Richter JE. Esophageal dilation in eosinophilic esophagitis. Best Pract Res Clin Gastroenterol 2015;29(5):815–28.

# Pharmacologic Treatment of Eosinophilic Esophagitis
## An Update

Alain M. Schoepfer, MD[a],*, Alex Straumann, MD[b,c],
Ekaterina Safroneeva, PhD[d]

## KEYWORDS

- Eosinophilic esophagitis • Pharmacologic treatment • Budesonide • Fluticasone
- Proton pump inhibitors • Biologic therapy

## KEY POINTS

- Proton pump inhibitors are effective in about half of patients in bringing esophageal eosinophilia into remission.
- Swallowed topical corticosteroids, such as budesonide and fluticasone, are highly effective in bringing esophageal eosinophilia into remission and in improving eosinophilic esophagitis (EoE)-related symptoms.
- Antiallergic drugs (cromoglycate sodium, montelukast) have no effect on EoE-related symptoms and esophageal eosinophilia.
- Several biologic therapies are currently under evaluation.

Disclaimers: None.
Conflict of Interest: A. Schoepfer received consulting fees and/or speaker fees and/or research grants from AstraZeneca, AG, Switzerland; Aptalis Pharma, Inc; Dr. Falk Pharma, GmbH, Germany; GlaxoSmithKline, AG; Nestlé S. A., Switzerland; Receptos, Inc; and Regeneron Pharmaceuticals. A. Straumann received consulting fees and/or speaker fees and/or research grants from Actelion, AG, Switzerland; AstraZeneca, AG, Switzerland; Adare Pharma, Inc; Dr. Falk Pharma, GmbH, Germany; Glaxo Smith Kline, AG; Nestlé S. A., Switzerland; Novartis, AG, Switzerland; Pfizer, AG, and Regeneron Pharmaceuticals, Inc. E. Safroneeva received consulting fees from Aptalis Pharma, Inc; and Novartis, AG, Switzerland.
Writing Assistance: None.
Grant Support: This work was supported by a grant from the Swiss National Science Foundation (grant no. 32473B_160115) and a grant from TIGERS (The International Gastrointestinal Eosinophil ResearcherS).
[a] Division of Gastroenterology and Hepatology, Centre Hospitalier Universitaire Vaudois (CHUV), Rue de Bugnon 44, 07/2409, Lausanne 1011, Switzerland; [b] Swiss EoE Clinic, Römerstrasse 7, 4600 Olten, Switzerland; [c] Division of Gastroenterology and Hepatology, Department of Internal Medicine, University Hospital Zurich, Rämistrasse 100, 8091 Zürich, Switzerland; [d] Institute of Social and Preventive Medicine, University of Bern, Finkenhubelweg 11, 3012 Bern, Switzerland
* Corresponding author.
E-mail address: alain.schoepfer@chuv.ch

Gastrointest Endoscopy Clin N Am 28 (2018) 77–88
http://dx.doi.org/10.1016/j.giec.2017.07.007

## INTRODUCTION
### Definition of Eosinophilic Esophagitis

The first consecutive case series of patients with eosinophilic esophagitis (EoE) were published in 1993 and 1994 by Dr Attwood and colleagues[1] and Dr Straumann and colleagues.[2] These described patients who were characterized by dysphagia and dense esophageal eosinophilic infiltration. In 2007, an international expert panel published the first guidelines on the diagnosis and therapy for EoE.[3] EoE is currently defined as a chronic, immune/antigen-mediated esophageal disease, characterized clinically by symptoms related to esophageal dysfunction and histologically by eosinophil-predominant inflammation.[4,5] This definition highlights that there is no single test to definitively diagnose EoE and that the diagnosis relies on a combination of typical symptoms and characteristic histologic findings.[6,7] EoE patients are mostly men and a high prevalence of allergies to inhaled or food antigens is observed.[8] Symptoms, mostly dysphagia, are typically present for years before EoE diagnosis is established.[9]

### Pathophysiology and Natural History of Eosinophilic Esophagitis

Knowledge of the pathophysiology of EoE is important to understand the treatment indications and the different treatment options. Unfortunately, the pathogenesis of EoE is still incompletely understood.[7] It is generally accepted that EoE results from a complex interplay between genetic, environmental, and host immune system factors.[7] Some researchers reported on esophageal barrier defects that might facilitate the entry of food allergens or swallowed aeroallergens into the esophageal epithelium. Rothenberg and colleagues[10] published on cadherins, a group of junctional proteins within the desmosomes; in particular, on the adhesion molecule desmoglein-1 (DSG1). They found that, when compared with controls, DSG1 is more than 20 times downregulated in active EoE and that DSG1 deficiency leads to a structural alteration of the esophageal epithelium. Other researchers found that, in pediatric patients with active EoE, the expression of the intercellular junction proteins E-cadherin and claudin-1 is reduced.[11] As such, mucosal integrity in active EoE is altered due to defects in tight junction adhesion proteins and desmosomal proteins. However, these functional defects are reversed by anti-inflammatory treatment of EoE, and the function of the mucosal barrier of patients having remittent EoE and of healthy controls is almost comparable.[11] These findings support that disturbed mucosal integrity in EoE is the result, and not the cause, of the chronic eosinophil inflammation.

Antigenic proteins, which are typically derived from food, can trigger an adaptive T helper 2 (Th2) cell–mediated response that produces a set of different cytokines, such as interleukin-5 (IL-5) and interleukin-13 (IL-13). IL-13 subsequently triggers esophageal resident cells, such as the epithelial cells, to produce a large set of proteins. Thymic stromal lymphopoietin promotes dendritic cell-mediated Th2 differentiation, whereas tumor necrosis factor alpha (TNFα) increases adhesion molecules on endothelial cells. The protein eotaxin-3 is strongly expressed by the esophageal epithelium and recruits eosinophils from the peripheral blood into the tissue.[12] Antigen-driven Th2 cells also produce IL-5, which activates eosinophils, enhances their responsiveness to eotaxin-3, and prolongs their survival. Eosinophils, T cells, and mast cells are elevated in esophageal mucosal biopsies with T cells being polarized toward aTh2 immunity.[13] A recent publication highlighted a potential role for immunoglobulin (Ig)G4 in EoE pathogenesis.[14] The production of transforming growth factor beta (TGFβ) by eosinophils leads to subepithelial fibrosis.[15] Knowledge of the key interleukins involved in EoE pathogenesis is important to appreciate the targets for biologic therapies.

There is now solid evidence that EoE is a chronic progressive disease that can lead, if eosinophil-predominant inflammation remains untreated, to esophageal remodeling processes with fibrous tissue deposition and resultant stricture formation.[16–20] The presence of esophageal strictures represents the key risk factor for feared food bolus impactions.[21,22] It is important to point out that the natural history of EoE is not characterized by a march from an inflammatory to a stricturing phenotype. Instead, in the absence of anti-inflammatory therapies, inflammatory activity continues and fibrotic features are added on top of ongoing inflammation.[20] The natural history of untreated EoE is not only characterized by morphologic alterations, such as esophageal strictures and histologically subepithelial fibrosis, but also functional abnormalities of esophageal motility.[23]

### Reasons to Treat Active Eosinophilic Esophagitis

EoE is a chronic and progressive disease. When pharmacologic or dietary treatments for EoE are stopped, symptoms and/or esophageal eosinophilia typically recur over 3 to 6 months.[5] There are several reasons to treat active EoE. First, to reduce EoE-related symptoms and to improve EoE-related quality of life.[24,25] Second, in the long-term, to reduce or prevent esophageal remodeling processes that are associated with stricture formation and food bolus impactions.[16–22]

### How to Assess the Efficacy of a Pharmacologic Treatment

Activity of EoE can be assessed by patient-reported outcomes (PROs) and clinician-reported outcomes (ClinROs).[26,27] PRO encompasses different domains of patient's self-reports, such as symptoms, disease-specific quality of life, general quality of life, disability, health status, and general health perceptions. PRO instruments that assess symptoms focus on particular disease-related impairments. The term disability describes activities, such as locomotor functioning, activities of daily living, and personal care. Health-specific quality of life questionnaires measure impairments and/or disability related to specific health problems inherent to a particular disease.[28] Disease-specific quality of life questionnaires benchmark health status based on items that are relevant to patient's perception of health. In contrast to health-specific quality of life, the general quality of life questionnaires assess the patient's ability to fulfill their needs and inquire about their emotional response to their restrictions.

ClinRO measures in EoE include assessment of histologic, endoscopic, and laboratory findings. Structural esophageal abnormalities may be detected by the means of endoluminal functional lumen imaging probe that measures esophageal caliper and wall distensibility.[29]

In EoE, both PRO and ClinRO measure disease activity.[26] As such, most clinical trials assess both PRO and ClinRO (eg, histology and endoscopy) to get a global view of EoE activity. Currently, there is no pharmacologic treatment specifically for EoE that is granted approval from regulatory authorities.

## THERAPEUTIC OPTIONS FOR EOSINOPHILIC ESOPHAGITIS

The therapy options to treat EoE can be summarized as the 3 Ds: drugs, diet, and dilation. For an in-depth review of therapy recommendations regarding the use of elimination diets and drug therapy, as well as esophageal dilation, please refer to evidence-based statements and recommendations for diagnosis and management in children and adults.[5] This article focuses on pharmacologic treatment options and does not discuss dietary strategies nor esophageal dilation. In clinical practice, the therapy choice strongly depends on the EoE phenotype (purely inflammatory features vs fibrotic features, or a combination of both), the disease impact as perceived by the patient, and patient preferences. Dietary therapy may represent an interesting nonpharmacologic option in patients not willing to undergo a pharmacologic treatment. The assets and shortcomings of the different therapeutic regimens are highlighted in **Table 1**.

The following pharmacologic treatment options exist for EoE: proton pump inhibitors (PPIs) and swallowed topical glucocorticoids, such as budesonide, fluticasone propionate, and ciclesonide. Antiallergic drugs, such as cromoglycate sodium and antihistamines, have been shown not to affect the histologic and clinical outcomes in EoE. Several biologic therapies have been and are currently being evaluated. The following section highlights the current evidence to support the use of the different pharmacologic regimens for EoE treatment.

### Proton Pump Inhibitors

Gastroesophageal reflux disease (GERD) may mimic, coexist, or contribute to EoE.[30] On the other hand, EoE can also contribute to GERD because it may affect the esophageal clearance.[31] EoE diagnosis is based on the persistence of esophageal eosinophilia despite a 2-month treatment with PPI or a normal pH-metric study.[5,6] PPI-therapy may benefit patients with coexistent GERD by reducing acid production or by PPI-inherent antieosinophil mechanisms.[32] PPI-therapy may also be helpful in patients with established EoE because the altered esophagus may be predisposed and more sensitive to physiologic acid exposure.[33] In fact, a recently published systematic review with meta-analysis that included 33 studies with 619 subjects showed that PPI led to histologic remission (<15 eosinophils/high-power field [HPF])

**Table 1**
**Advantages and shortcomings of different established therapeutic options for treatment of eosinophilic esophagitis**

| Modality | Advantages | Shortcomings |
|---|---|---|
| Drugs | | |
| Proton pump inhibitors (PPIs) | • Good histologic and clinical efficacy<br>• Rarely side effects<br>• No dietary restriction necessary | • No data regarding effect on fibrosis<br>• Limited long-term data |
| Swallowed topical steroids | • Good histologic and clinical efficacy<br>• No dietary restriction necessary<br>• Antifibrotic effect | • Limited data regarding long-term safety |
| Biologic therapies | • Pharmacologic option for patients unresponsive to PPI and swallowed topical corticosteroids | • Costs<br>• Availability<br>• Limited data regarding efficacy |
| Elimination diets | • Nonpharmacologic approach<br>• Good histologic and clinical efficacy<br>• Antifibrotic effect | • Repetitive upper endoscopy necessary to identify offending food<br>• Needs motivated patient |
| Esophageal dilation | • Long-lasting symptom improvement<br>• Safe procedure | • No influence on underlying inflammation<br>• Postprocedural thoracic pain (temporarily) |

in 50.5% (95% CI 42.2%–58.7%) and symptomatic improvement in 60.8% (95% CI 48.4%–72.2%) of subjects.[34] The investigators detected no significant differences in subjects' age, study design, and type of PPI used.[34] They observed a trend for increased clinicohistologic efficacy when PPIs were given twice daily compared with once daily and in patients with a pathologic pH monitoring.[34] Of note, the investigators offered a word of caution regarding the interpretation of their findings due to poor-quality evidence (mostly case reports and retrospective studies, with no placebo-controlled trials), heterogeneity in results, and publication bias in favor of studies reporting histologic responses to PPI.

There is increasing evidence that PPIs are not only effective in inducing clinical and histologic responses but also in maintaining them. A recently published prospective study in a pediatric cohort showed that most PPI-responsive esophageal eosinophilia (PPI-REE) subjects (78%) remained in clinicopathologic remission at the 1-year follow-up on maintenance PPI therapy.[35] The first long-term follow-up multicenter study in 75 adult PPI-REE subjects revealed that all subjects who temporarily discontinued PPI therapy had a symptomatic and/or histologic relapse.[36] A total of 73% of subjects maintained histologic remission after at least 1 year when PPI dosages were tapered to the minimum effective clinical dose. Most subjects who relapsed regained histologic remission after dose escalation, which suggests that some patients might require high-dose PPI therapy long-term.[36] Of note, there are no data available yet regarding the clinicohistological efficacy of PPI for follow-up longer than 1 year.

### Swallowed Topical Corticosteroids: Budesonide, Fluticasone Propionate, Ciclesonide

There are currently 12 randomized clinical trials in pediatric and adult subjects that have confirmed the efficacy of swallowed topical corticosteroids (budesonide and fluticasone propionate) to induce histologic remission in subjects with histologically active EoE.[37–48] The results of these trials have been summarized in several systematic reviews and meta-analyses.[49–52] Systematic reviews described considerable variability of different trials with respect to inclusion criteria, drugs evaluated (budesonide, fluticasone propionate), daily dosages, delivery system (suspension, viscous slurry, swallowed puffs from inhalers, effervescent tablets), and the definition of histologic remission (ranges from <1–<20 eosinophils/HPF), which hinders the comparison between the different studies. For a comparative analysis of different dosages used in the various studies, please refer to the recently published EoE guidelines.[5] In 2012, Dellon and colleagues[45] showed for the first time that a topical steroid delivery that enhances esophageal mucosal contact time, such as viscous slurry, is more effective regarding histologic response compared with the swallowing of a nebulized steroid. A recently published meta-analysis and systematic review showed that higher rates of histologic remission were achieved by effervescent tablets and oral viscous budesonide.[52] One trial with 4 children evaluated ciclesonide, a topical glucocorticoid with less systemic absorption than fluticasone and showed that symptoms, as well as eosinophil counts, significantly decreased after 2 months of treatment.[53]

Besides histologic response and remission, the improvement of EoE-related symptoms represents another important therapeutic endpoint.[54] Until recently, data on symptomatic improvement were less clear than data on histologic improvement. Two recently published meta-analyses did not observe a clear trend in symptomatic improvement in EoE subjects using swallowed topical corticosteroids compared with placebo.[51,52] There are several reasons that explain this discrepancy between histologic and clinical outcomes, including differences in patient selection, differences in definitions of clinical response, different treatment durations, different steroid formulations, and the use of mostly nonvalidated scores to measure symptomatic activity.[51,52] Of note, assessment of dysphagia, the key symptom of adults with EoE, is complex because dysphagia frequency and severity depend on food consistency, as well as on behavioral modification strategies, such as food avoidance, food modification (eg, cutting meat in tiny pieces), and slow eating. There is now evidence that, when measuring symptomatic EoE activity using validated scores, such as the Dysphagia Symptom Questionnaire and the Eosinophilic Esophagitis Activity Index PRO instrument, histologic improvement is also correlated with symptom improvement.[48,55]

EoE is a chronic progressive disorder. As such, a long-term maintenance treatment is typically required. There is a paucity of studies evaluating the long-term efficacy of swallowed topical steroids in pediatric and adult EoE subjects.[56] One randomized, double-blind, placebo-controlled trial evaluated the efficacy of swallowed topical budesonide suspension with 0.5 mg/d versus placebo for a duration of 50 weeks. Histologic remission, defined as less than 5 eosinophils per HPF, was found in 36% of subjects in the budesonide group, whereas no subject in the placebo group remained in remission. It is possible that the maintenance dosage of budesonide was too low. An open-label, prospective, single-center study in children offered age-dependent dosages of swallowed topical fluticasone from metered-dose inhalers and showed, over a mean follow-up time of 24 months, an improvement with respect to histology, endoscopy, and symptoms.[57]

With regard to safety aspects, the use of swallowed topical steroids in the short-term and long-term run seems to have a favorable safety profile with no serious side effects reported. Esophageal candidiasis is observed in up to 10% of subjects, which represents a mostly incidental finding.[52] There remains some uncertainty regarding suppression of systemic cortisol levels induced by swallowed topical corticosteroids. In clinical trials evaluating induction treatment with swallowed topical steroids, the 24-hour urine and/or serum cortisol levels were not suppressed.[46,47] There are conflicting results regarding the long-term use of swallowed topical steroids and their impact on adrenal suppression, particularly in children. Philla and colleagues[58] detected, in 14 children, no differences in serum cortisol levels following treatment with swallowed fluticasone propionate (range 220–880 µg/d) and budesonide (range 0.5–1 mg/d) for a treatment duration of 8 to 43 weeks. Golekoh and colleagues,[59] however, documented adrenal suppression in 10% of children treated with swallowed topical steroids for 6 or more months. No symptoms of adrenal insufficiency or impaired growth were reported so far.[58]

### Systemic Steroids

Systemic steroids are not recommended to be used in EoE given their side-effect profile and the generally high efficacy of topical swallowed steroids.[5] One randomized trial evaluated oral prednisolone versus swallowed topical fluticasone.[44] At week 4, almost all subjects, irrespective of the treatment group, were free of symptoms, whereas histologic improvement was noted to be greater in the prednisone group. As expected, glucocorticoid side effects were more frequently observed in the prednisone group compared with the fluticasone group.[60]

### Azathioprine and Mercaptopurine

One case series with 3 subjects documented a clinical and histologic response to azathioprine or 6-mercaptopurine in steroid-dependent EoE subjects.[60] As such, azathioprine and 6-mercaptopurine might have a role in inducing and maintaining long-term clinical and histologic remission in EoE in limited cases. One factor limiting the wide-spread use of these drugs is their side-effect profile.[61]

### Antiallergic Drugs: Sodium Cromoglycate and Antihistamines

Several antiallergic drugs were evaluated for EoE treatment but failed to show a clinically relevant improvement on either histologic activity and EoE-related symptoms.

A 4-week trial of the mast cell stabilizer sodium cromoglycate failed to show either symptomatic or histologic improvement in 14 children with EoE.[62]

Montelukast is a leukotriene D4 receptor antagonist. In open-labeled trials, its use in high doses in adults and standard doses in children led, to a certain extent, to symptomatic improvement but failed to demonstrate a histologic response.[63,64] In a randomized controlled trial, Alexander and colleagues[65] found that montelukast (20 mg/d) was not superior to placebo to maintain remission induced by swallowed topical steroids. Similarly, montelukast failed to maintain remission induced by swallowed topical steroids in a prospective study in adult EoE subjects, with reappearance of symptoms and histologic inflammation within 3 months.[66]

One randomized, double-blind, placebo-controlled study evaluated the efficacy of the oral prostaglandin D2 receptor antagonist OC000459.[67] A total of 26 adult subjects with steroid-dependent or steroid-refractory EoE were randomized to either receive OC000459 or placebo. At week 8, OC000459 but not placebo was associated with a significant reduction in esophageal eosinophil counts and an improvement in symptoms; however, no normalization of esophageal biopsies was documented.[68]

### Biological Drugs

Several biological agents have been and are currently evaluated for use in active EoE.

Mepolizumab and reslizumab are both anti–IL-5 monoclonal antibodies that have been evaluated in 3 randomized, double-blind, placebo-controlled trials in children, adolescents, and adults with EoE.[67,69,70] All 3 trials showed a significant reduction of esophageal eosinophilic infiltrations; however, histologic remission was not observed. An improvement of EoE-related symptoms was found in 2 studies.[69,71]

QAX576 is an anti–IL-13 antibody that was evaluated in a randomized, double-blind, placebo-controlled trial in adults with EoE. QAX576 reduced the mean peak eosinophil count by 60%; however, no improvement was noted with respect to symptoms.[71] Other anti–IL-13 antibodies are currently under evaluation.

Omalizumab is a monoclonal anti–IgE antibody. A randomized, double-blind, placebo-controlled trial in adult EoE subjects showed no benefits compared with placebo with respect to esophageal eosinophil counts and EoE-related symptoms.[14]

Infliximab is a monoclonal antibody against TNF$\alpha$, which was evaluated in a dose of 5 mg/kg body weight in 3 adult EoE subjects. An induction treatment at weeks 0, 2, and 6, did not lead to an improvement of EoE-related symptoms and esophageal eosinophilia. Other monoclonal antibodies against TNF$\alpha$, such as adalimumab or golimumab have not been evaluated in EoE patients.

### SUMMARY

Although the first EoE patients were described only a little more than 20 years ago, considerable progress has been made in evaluating different treatment options, as well as in understanding the pathophysiology and the natural history. Therapeutic options in EoE include drugs, elimination diets, and esophageal dilation. Regarding drugs, PPIs and swallowed topical corticosteroids (budesonide or fluticasone propionate) represent the most frequently used drugs in active EoE with proven efficacy in inducing clinical and histologic response and remission. PPI, as well as swallowed topical steroids, have a favorable safety profile. In the near future, swallowed topical steroids will probably be the first drugs on the market that receive approval from regulatory authorities. Systemic steroids are rarely used to treat active EoE and have a high prevalence of systemic side effects. There is limited evidence that azathioprine and mercaptopurine can induce and maintain long-term histologic and clinical remission in patients with steroid-resistant disease. Antiallergic drugs, such as cromoglycate sodium, montelukast, and OC000459 (an oral selective antagonist of CRTH2) did not show an effect on symptoms and histology. Several biologic therapies have been evaluated and have shown potential to improve histologic outcomes, whereas the effect on EoE-related symptoms remains less clear. Other biologic therapies are currently under evaluation. Long-term safety data with the different drugs are currently lacking. Concerted efforts of different stakeholders are necessary to continue the endeavor of providing patients with much-needed therapies.

## REFERENCES

1. Attwood SE, Smyrk TC, Demeester TR, et al. Esophageal eosinophilia with dysphagia, a distinct clinicopathologic syndrome. Dig Dis Sci 1993;38:109–16.
2. Straumann A, Spichtin HP, Bernoulli R, et al. Idiopathic eosinophilic esophagitis: a frequently overlooked disease with typical clinical aspects and discrete endoscopic findings. Schweiz Med Wochenschr 1994;124:1419–29 [in German with English abstract].
3. Furuta GT, Liacouras CA, Collins MH, et al. Eosinophilic esophagitis in children and adults: a systematic review and consensus recommendations for diagnosis and treatment. Gastroenterology 2007;133:1342–63.
4. Liacouras CA, Furuta GT, Hirano I, et al. Eosinophilic esophagitis: updated consensus recommendations for children and adults. J Allergy Clin Immunol 2011;128:3–20.
5. Lucendo AJ, Molina-Infante J, Arias A, et al. Guidelines on eosinophilic esophagitis: evidence-based statements and recommendations for diagnosis and management in children and adults. United European Gastroenterol J 2017;5:335–58.
6. Dellon ES, Gonsalves N, Hirano I, et al. ACG clinical guideline: evidenced based approach to the diagnosis and management of esophageal eosinophilia and eosinophilic esophagitis (EoE). Am J Gastroenterol 2013;108:679–92.
7. Furuta GT, Katzka DA. Eosinophilic esophagitis. N Engl J Med 2015;373:1640–8.
8. Spergel JM, Brown-Whitehorn T, Beausoleil JL, et al. Predictive values for skin prick test and atopy patch test for eosinophilic esophagitis. J Allergy Clin Immunol 2007;119:509–11.
9. Straumann A, Spichtin HP, Grize L, et al. Natural history of primary eosinophilic esophagitis: a follow-up of 30 adult patients for up to 11.5 years. Gastroenterology 2003;125:1660–9.
10. Sherrill JD, Kc K, Wu D, et al. Desmoglein-1 regulates esophageal epithelial barrier function and immune responses in eosinophilic esophagitis. Mucosal Immunol 2014;7:718–29.
11. Abdulnour-Nakhoul SM, Al-Tawil Y, Gyftopoulos AA, et al. Alterations in junctional proteins, inflammatory mediators and extracellular matrix molecules in eosinophilic esophagitis. Clin Immunol 2013;148:265–78.
12. Hogan SP, Mishra A, Brandt EB, et al. A critical role for eotaxin in experimental oral antigen-induced eosinophilic gastrointestinal allergy. Proc Natl Acad Sci U S A 2000;97:6681–6.
13. Straumann A, Bauer M, Fischer B, et al. Idiopathic eosinophilic esophagitis is associated with a T(H)2-type allergic inflammatory response. J Allergy Clin Immunol 2001;108:954–61.

14. Clayton F, Fang JC, Gleich GJ, et al. Eosinophilic esophagitis in adults is associated with IgG4 and not mediated by IgE. Gastroenterology 2014;147:602–9.
15. Straumann A, Aceves SS, Blanchard C, et al. Pediatric and adult eosinophilic esophagitis: similarities and differences. Allergy 2012;67:477–90.
16. Assa'ad AH, Putnam PE, Collins MH, et al. Pediatric patients with eosinophilic esophagitis: an 8-year follow-up. J Allergy Clin Immunol 2007;119:731–8.
17. Helou EF, Simonson J, Arora AS. 3-yr-follow-up of topical corticosteroid treatment for eosinophilic esophagitis in adults. Am J Gastroenterol 2008;103:2194–9.
18. Spergel JM, Brown-Whitehorn TF, Beausoleil JL, et al. 14 years of eosinophilic esophagitis: clinical features and prognosis. J Pediatr Gastroenterol Nutr 2009; 48:30–6.
19. Kagalwalla AF, Akhtar N, Woodruff SA, et al. Eosinophilic esophagitis: epithelial mesenchymal transition contributes to esophageal remodeling and reverses with treatment. J Allergy Clin Immunol 2012;129:1387–96.
20. Schoepfer AM, Safroneeva E, Bussmann C, et al. Delay in diagnosis of eosinophilic esophagitis increases risk for stricture formation in a time-dependent manner. Gastroenterology 2013;145:1230–6.
21. Lipka S, Kumar A, Richter JE. Impact of diagnostic delay and other risk factors on eosinophilic esophagitis phenotype and esophageal diameter. J Clin Gastroenterol 2016;50:134–40.
22. Dellon ES, Kim HP, Sperry SL, et al. A phenotypic analysis shows that eosinophilic esophagitis is a progressive fibrostenotic disease. Gastrointest Endosc 2014;79: 577–85.
23. Van Rhijn BD, Oors JM, Smout AJ, et al. Prevalence of esophageal motility abnormalities increases with longer disease duration in adult patients with eosinophilic esophagitis. Neurogastroenterol Motil 2014;26:1349–55.
24. Taft TH, Kern E, Kwiatek MA, et al. The adult eosinophilic oesophagitis quality of life questionnaire: a new measure of health-related quality of life. Aliment Pharmacol Ther 2011;34:790–8.
25. Safroneeva E, Coslovsky M, Kuehni CE, et al. Eosinophilic oesophagitis: relationship of quality of life with clinical, endoscopic and histological activity. Aliment Pharmacol Ther 2015;42:1000–10.
26. Schoepfer AM, Hirano I, Katzka DA. Eosinophilic esophagitis: overview of clinical management. Gastroenterol Clin North Am 2014;43:329–44.
27. Schoepfer A, Safroneeva E, Straumann A. How to measure disease activity in eosinophilic esophagitis. Dis Esophagus 2016;29:959–66.
28. Guyatt GH, Feeny DH, Patrick DL. Measuring health-related quality of life. Ann Intern Med 1993;118:622–9.
29. Kwiatek MA, Hirano I, Kahrilas PJ, et al. Mechanical properties of the esophagus in eosinophilic esophagitis. Gastroenterology 2011;140:82–90.
30. Remedios M, Campbell C, Jones DM, et al. Eosinophilic esophagitis in adults: clinical, endoscopic, histologic findings, and response to treatment with fluticasone propionate. Gastrointest Endosc 2006;63:3–12.
31. Spechler SJ, Genta RM, Souza RF. Thoughts on the complex relationship between gastroesophageal reflux disease and eosinophilic esophagitis. Am J Gastroenterol 2007;102:1301–6.
32. Cheng E, Zhang X, Huo X, et al. Omeprazole blocks eotaxin-3 expression by oesophageal squamous cells from patients with eosinophilic oesophagitis and GORD. Gut 2013;62:824–32.
33. Krarup AL, Villadsen GE, Mejlgaard E, et al. Acid hypersensitivity in patients with eosinophilic oesophagitis. Scand J Gastroenterol 2010;45:273–81.

34. Lucendo AJ, Arias Á, Molina-Infante J. Efficacy of proton pump inhibitor drugs for inducing clinical and histologic remission in patients with symptomatic esophageal eosinophilia: a systematic review and meta-analysis. Clin Gastroenterol Hepatol 2016;14:13–22.

35. Gutierrez-Junquera C, Fernandez-Fernandez S, Cilleruelo ML, et al. High prevalence of response to proton-pump inhibitor treatment in children with esophageal eosinophilia. J Pediatr Gastroenterol Nutr 2016;62:704–10.

36. Molina-Infante J, Rodriguez-Sanchez J, Martinek J, et al. Long-term loss of response in proton pump inhibitor-responsive esophageal eosinophilia is uncommon and influenced by CYP2C19 genotype and rhinoconjunctivitis. Am J Gastroenterol 2015;110:1567–75.

37. Straumann A, Conus S, Degen L, et al. Budesonide is effective in adolescent and adult patients with active eosinophilic esophagitis. Gastroenterology 2010;139: 1526–37.

38. Alexander JA, Jung KW, Arora AS, et al. Swallowed fluticasone improves histologic but not symptomatic response of adults with eosinophilic esophagitis. Clin Gastroenterol Hepatol 2012;10:742–9.

39. Dohil R, Newbury R, Fox L, et al. Oral viscous budesonide is effective in children with eosinophilic esophagitis in a randomized, placebo-controlled trial. Gastroenterology 2010;139:418–29.

40. Gupta SK, Vitanza JM, Collins MH. Efficacy and safety of oral budesonide suspension in pediatric patients with eosinophilic esophagitis. Clin Gastroenterol Hepatol 2015;13:66–76.

41. Peterson KA, Thomas KL, Hilden K, et al. Comparison of esomeprazole to aerosolized, swallowed fluticasone for eosinophilic esophagitis. Dig Dis Sci 2010;55: 1313–9.

42. Moawad FJ, Veerappan GR, Dias JA, et al. Randomized controlled trial comparing aerosolized swallowed fluticasone to esomeprazole for esophageal eosinophilia. Am J Gastroenterol 2013;108:366–72.

43. Konikoff MR, Noel RJ, Blanchard C, et al. A randomized, double-blind, placebo-controlled trial of fluticasone propionate for pediatric eosinophilic esophagitis. Gastroenterology 2006;131:1381–91.

44. Schaefer ET, Fitzgerald JF, Molleston JP, et al. Comparison of oral prednisone and topical fluticasone in the treatment of eosinophilic esophagitis: a randomized trial in children. Clin Gastroenterol Hepatol 2008;6:165–73.

45. Dellon ES, Sheikh A, Speck O, et al. Viscous topical is more effective than nebulized steroid therapy for patients with eosinophilic esophagitis. Gastroenterology 2012;143:321–4.

46. Butz BK, Wen T, Gleich GJ, et al. Efficacy, dose reduction, and resistance to high-dose fluticasone in patients with eosinophilic esophagitis. Gastroenterology 2014;147:324–33.

47. Miehlke S, Hruz P, Vieth M, et al. A randomised, double-blind trial comparing budesonide formulations and dosages for short-term treatment of eosinophilic oesophagitis. Gut 2016;65:390–9.

48. Dellon ES, Katzka DA, Collins MH, et al. Budesonide oral suspension improves symptomatic, endoscopic, and histologic parameters compared with placebo in patients with eosinophilic esophagitis. Gastroenterology 2017;152:776–86.

49. Sawas T, Dhalla S, Sayyar M, et al. Systematic review with meta-analysis: pharmacological interventions for eosinophilic oesophagitis. Aliment Pharmacol Ther 2015;41:797–806.

50. Tan ND, Xiao YL, Chen MH. Steroids therapy for eosinophilic esophagitis: systematic review and meta-analysis. J Dig Dis 2015;16:431–42.

51. Murali AR, Gupta A, Attar BM, et al. Topical steroids in eosinophilic esophagitis: systematic review and meta-analysis of placebo controlled randomized clinical trials. J Gastroenterol Hepatol 2015;31:1111–9.

52. Chuang MYA, Chinnaratha MA, Hancock DG, et al. Topical steroid therapy for the treatment of eosinophilic esophagitis (EoE): a systematic review and metaanalysis. Clin Transl Gastroenterol 2015;6:e82.

53. Schroeder S, Fleischer DM, Masterson JC, et al. Successful treatment of eosinophilic esophagitis with ciclesonide. J Allergy Clin Immunol 2012;129:1419–21.

54. Hirano I. Therapeutic end points in eosinophilic esophagitis: is elimination of esophageal eosinophils enough? Clin Gastroenterol Hepatol 2012;10:750–2.

55. Lucendo A, Miehlke S, Vieth M, et al. Budesonide or dispersible tablets are highly effective for treatment of active eosinophilic esophagitis: results from a randomized, double-blind, placebo-controlled, pivotal multicenter trial (EOS-1) [abstract]. Gastroenterology 2017;152(Suppl 1):A1118. S207.

56. Straumann A, Conus S, Degen L, et al. Long-term budesonide maintenance treatment is partially effective for patients with eosinophilic esophagitis. Clin Gastroenterol Hepatol 2011;9:400–9.

57. Andreae DA, Hanna MG, Magid MS, et al. Swallowed fluticasone propionate is an effective long-term maintenance therapy for children with eosinophilic esophagitis. Am J Gastroenterol 2016;111:1187–97.

58. Philla KQ, Min SB, Hefner JN, et al. Swallowed glucocorticoid therapy for eosinophilic esophagitis in children does not suppress adrenal function. J Pediatr Endocrinol Metab 2015;28:1101–6.

59. Golekoh MC, Hornung LN, Mukkada VA, et al. Adrenal insufficiency after chronic swallowed glucocorticoid therapy for eosinophilic esophagitis. J Pediatr 2016; 170:240–5.

60. Netzer P, Gschossmann JM, Straumann A, et al. Corticosteroid-dependent eosinophilic esophagitis: azathioprine and 6-mercaptopurine can induce and maintain long-term remission. Eur J Gastroenterol Hepatol 2007;19:865–9.

61. Mottet C, Schoepfer AM, Juillerat P, et al. Experts opinion on the practical use of azathioprine and 6-mercaptopurine in inflammatory bowel disease. Inflamm Bowel Dis 2016;22:2733–47.

62. Liacouras CA, Spergel JM, Ruchelli E, et al. Eosinophilic esophagitis: a 10-year experience in 381 children. Clin Gastroenterol Hepatol 2005;3:1198–206.

63. Attwood SEA, Lewis CJ, Bronder CS, et al. Eosinophilic oesophagitis: a novel treatment using Montelukast. Gut 2003;52:181–5.

64. Stumphy J, Al-Zubeidi D, Guerin L, et al. Observations on use of montelukast in pediatric eosinophilic esophagitis: insights for the future. Dis Esophagus 2011; 24:229–34.

65. Alexander JA, Ravi K, Enders FT, et al. Montelukast does not maintain symptom reductions following topical steroid therapy for eosinophilic esophagitis. Clin Gastroenterol Hepatol 2017;15:214–21.

66. Lucendo AJ, De Rezende LC, Jimenez-Contreras S, et al. Montelukast was inefficient in maintaining steroid-induced remission in adult eosinophilic esophagitis. Dig Dis Sci 2011;56:3551–8.

67. Straumann A, Conus S, Grzonka P, et al. Anti-interleukin-5 antibody treatment (mepolizumab) in active eosinophilic oesophagitis: a randomised, placebo-controlled, double-blind trial. Gut 2010;59:21–30.

68. Straumann A, Hoesli S, Bussmann C, et al. Anti-eosinophil activity and clinical efficacy of the CRTH2 antagonist OC000459 in eosinophilic esophagitis. Allergy 2013;68:375–85.

69. Assa'ad AH, Gupta SK, Collins MH, et al. An antibody against IL-5 reduces numbers of esophageal intraepithelial eosinophils in children with eosinophilic esophagitis. Gastroenterology 2011;141:1593–604.

70. Spergel JM, Rothenberg ME, Collins MH, et al. Reslizumab in children and adolescents with eosinophilic esophagitis: results of a double-blind, randomized, placebo-controlled trial. J Allergy Clin Immunol 2012;129:456–63.

71. Rothenberg ME, Wen T, Greenberg A, et al. Intravenous anti-IL-13 mAb QAX576 for the treatment of eosinophilic esophagitis. J Allergy Clin Immunol 2015;135: 500–7.

# Dietary Therapy in Eosinophilic Esophagitis

Nirmala Gonsalves, MD

## KEYWORDS

- Dietary therapy • Eosinophilic esophagitis • Dysphagia

## KEY POINTS

- The effectiveness of dietary elimination therapy in adults supports the concept that the pathophysiology driving eosinophilic esophagitis (EoE) is similar in children and adults, with food antigens as the main environmental trigger.
- Optimization and personalization of dietary therapy may be possible with a more tailored approach to dietary therapy and elimination of few antigens to achieve remission.
- Both medical and dietary therapy are effective in treating EoE in adults and children and choosing the right treatment should take into consideration both patient goals and available resources.

## INTRODUCTION

Recent consensus guidelines define eosinophilic esophagitis (EoE) as a chronic, immune-mediated or antigen-mediated esophageal disease characterized clinically by symptoms related to esophageal dysfunction and histologically by eosinophil (eos)-predominant inflammation.[1] In adults, the most common presenting symptoms include dysphagia and food impaction, whereas symptoms in children may include these in addition to reflux, heartburn, regurgitation, nausea and vomiting, feeding difficulties, and failure to thrive.[1,2] The concept of food allergens as the main antigenic trigger in EoE was introduced in a landmark study by Kelly and Sampson in pediatric subjects with symptoms of gastroesophageal reflux disease and histologic features of esophageal eosinophilia, both of which were unresponsive to acid suppression or fundoplication surgery.[3] After treatment with an elemental or amino acid–based formula, both symptoms and histologic eosinophilia resolved.[3,4] Since this landmark study, numerous series have replicated this association of food allergens as a trigger in EoE in the adult and pediatric population.[5–9] Common food triggers found to cause EoE in children and adults include milk, wheat, soy, egg, nuts or peanuts, and fish or shellfish.[6,9]

Division of Gastroenterology and Hepatology, Northwestern University Feinberg School of Medicine, 676 North St Clair Street, Suite 1400, Chicago, IL 60611-2951, USA
*E-mail address:* n-gonsalves@northwestern.edu

Gastrointest Endoscopy Clin N Am 28 (2018) 89–96
http://dx.doi.org/10.1016/j.giec.2017.07.008
1052-5157/18/© 2017 Elsevier Inc. All rights reserved.

Optimal goals of treatment in EoE involve resolution of clinical symptoms, histologic inflammation and endoscopic abnormalities. Other important endpoints include prevention of complications of the disease, including fibrostenotic changes such as strictures, avoidance of food bolus impaction, and avoidance of esophageal perforation either spontaneously from retching during a food impaction or iatrogenically from stricture dilation. Improvement in patients' quality of life and improvement of nutritional deficits are also important considerations in choosing a treatment modality. This article reviews current data and developments in the use of dietary therapy over the past year.

## DIETARY THERAPY IN EOSINOPHILIC ESOPHAGITIS

Dietary therapy has long been accepted as first-line therapy in children and was recently shown to be effective in adults.[7,10,11] Three approaches to dietary therapy in EoE have evolved. The first is complete elimination of all food allergens by placing patients on an elemental or amino acid–based formula as their primary source of nutrition. Patients are usually placed on this diet for at least 6 weeks followed by a reintroduction period to identify food culprits. Another approach to dietary therapy has been allergy-directed diets using the information gained from routine allergy testing to help guide the foods that are to be restricted. Although this has been shown to be helpful in some pediatric cohorts,[12] this has had limited utility in adult populations due to the lack of correlation with allergy testing and food triggers.[7,10,13] The last approach of empirical dietary elimination is the elimination of the 6 most likely food culprits, known as the 6-food elimination diet (SFED), which has been shown to be equally effective in children and adults.[5,7,14]

### Goals of Diet Therapy

Knowing that dietary therapy is effective in children and adults provides the rationale to offering this treatment approach as an alternative to swallowed topical corticosteroids. It is important to highlight that the goals of dietary therapy are not to stay on a restrictive diet indefinitely but rather to undergo a process of identifying food triggers to help tailor the diet for long-term maintenance therapy. Dietary elimination with food reintroduction has the ability to identify the actual food triggers of the disease. This treatment plan should be individualized based on each patient, their goals, and available resources at the treating center.

## RECENT LITERATURE
### Effectiveness of Elemental Diets in Adults

Although dietary therapy has been well established as an effective first-line therapy in pediatric patients for EoE, this approach has not been extensively used in adults. A prior study by Peterson and colleagues[11] evaluated the effectiveness of an elemental diet in a small group of adults. They found that 50% of adults responded histologically to the diet with less than 5 eos per high-power field (HPF) and 72% had less than 10 eos per HPF with eos levels dropping from 54 to 10, on average, after the diet. Interestingly, subjects did not demonstrate symptomatic improvement; however, that may be due to limitations in the dysphagia assessment tool used in this study and the presence of stricture formation. The investigators also suspect that decreased efficacy seen in this study compared with that of pediatric subjects might be attributed to adherence issues on the diet in their subject population. Another more recent study by Warners and colleagues[15] studied 21 adult subjects treated with 4 weeks of elemental diet. Of the 17 subjects who completed the diet, 12 (71%) showed complete histologic response, defined as less than 15 eos per HPF, and 4 (24%) showed partial histologic response (>50% reduction of baseline eos count). Responders to the diet experienced improvement in histologic inflammation, endoscopic signs, and symptoms. These investigators also showed improvement in esophageal and small intestinal mucosal integrity after treatment with the elemental diet. A recent meta-analysis performed by Lucendo[14] has also shown that elemental diet is the most effective approach (91%) in both children and adults. However, there are many practical limitations of this approach, including cost of the formula, palatability of the formula, and overall length of the food reintroduction period. Due to these limitations, elemental diet is not the favored approach in dietary therapy in adults.

### Effectiveness of Allergy-Directed Diets

One of the first studies to attempt a form of allergy-directed diets in adults was pursued in a small number of adult subjects in Switzerland by Simon and colleagues.[16] In this study, based on results of immunoglobulin E testing to certain foods, few foods were eliminated from the diet. Despite elimination of these foods, subjects did not respond symptomatically. The subject who completed endoscopic evaluation after dietary therapy also did not show histologic response. A more recent study undertaken by Molina-Infante and colleagues[13] studied the outcome of an allergy-directed diet using a multimodal approach, including skin prick testing, prick-prick testing, and atopy patch testing to identify allergens in their adult EoE cohort of 22 subjects. Disappointingly, they found only a 26% improvement with this approach. Likewise, allergy testing was not found to be predictive of food triggers in either the Gonsalves[7] or the Lucendo[10] study. A recent meta-analysis by Lucendo and colleagues[14] showed the efficacy of allergy-directed diets to be only 46%; therefore, current allergic testing methods are not reliable tools to guide dietary intervention in adults with EoE (**Fig. 1**).

### Effectiveness of Empiric Elimination Diets in Adults

Recently, empiric dietary elimination has been shown to have comparable effectiveness in adults and children. In a retrospective study, Kagalwalla and colleagues[5]

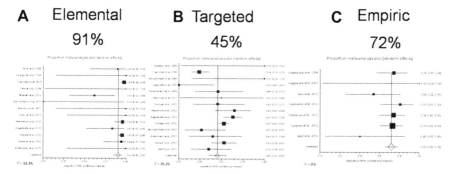

| A | Elemental | B | Targeted | C | Empiric |
| --- | --- | --- | --- | --- | --- |
| | 91% | | 45% | | 72% |

**Fig. 1.** (A) Summarized effects of elemental diets, (B) skin allergy testing–directed food removal, and (C) empirical SFED for inducing histologic remission of EoE, according to a recent meta-analysis.[14] Confidence intervals at 95% were calculated using the exact binomial method. $I^2$ values indicate the heterogeneity or intrastudy differences. The higher efficacy rate was for elemental diets (91%), followed by SFED, which showed a combined response rate of 72%, extremely homogeneous among the individual studies considered ($I^2 = 0\%$). Skin allergy testing–directed food removal showed the lowest combined effectiveness (45%) with a wide heterogeneity of results from individual studies. $I^2$, If P<.1 and/or $I^2$ >50%, there was significant heterogeneity and a random-effects model was used. Generally, $I^2$ was used to evaluate the level of heterogeneity, assigning the categories low, moderate, and high to $I^2$ values of 25%, 50% and 75% respectively.

demonstrated that the effectiveness of SFED (elimination of the 6 most common food allergens: wheat, milk, soy, egg, nuts, seafood) was 74%. During food reintroduction, the most common food triggers found in the pediatric group were milk, wheat, soy, and egg. Gonsalves and colleagues[7] prospectively studied the efficacy of this diet in 50 adults (25 men, 25 women) with EoE. Of these subjects, 70% had histologic response of less than 10 eos per HPF, 94% had symptomatic improvement, and 74% had endoscopic improvement after completing the diet for 6 weeks. Serial food reintroduction was undertaken in subjects who responded to the diet. When food triggers were identified, symptoms typically recurred within 5 days and esophageal eos counts returned to pretreatment values ($P<.0001$) on follow-up endoscopy. In this study, common food allergens identified during this process were wheat (60%), milk (50%), soy (10%), nuts (10%), and eggs (5%). Most subjects in this study had only a single food trigger. Allergy testing with skin prick testing was undertaken before the elimination diet but was predictive of food triggers in only 13% of cases.[7]

Since these studies, Lucendo and colleagues,[10] from Spain, demonstrated similar results in 67 adults with EoE after empiric elimination of wheat, rice, corn, legumes, peanuts, soy, egg, milk, fish, and shellfish for a similar duration. This approach resulted in histologic improvement of less than 15 eos per HPF in 73% of subjects but required additional foods to be removed. Food reintroduction in this study identified the common triggers as milk (61%), wheat (28%), eggs (26%), and legumes (23%). Unlike the prior study, most subjects in this study were found to have multiple food antigens as their trigger. A single offending food antigen was identified in only 36% of subjects. Two food triggers were found in 31% and 3 or more triggers were found in 33%. Results of allergy testing in this cohort of subjects were also not predictive of their food trigger. This group also found that continued elimination of these food triggers was effective in maintaining remission.

A meta-analysis looking at empirical elimination diet has shown efficacy of 76% using an empirical elimination approach.[14] Knowing that the common food triggers in all the studies tended to be milk, wheat, soy, and egg, tailored dietary elimination has also been undertaken. Kagalwalla and colleagues[17] investigated the utility of a single-food elimination diet in their subjects. In this retrospective study between 2006 and 2011, 17 subjects who had empirically eliminated cow's milk protein from the diet and had a follow-up endoscopy were included. Of these subjects, 65% achieved remission as defined by less than 15 eos per HPF after therapy. Although this study has encouraging results, further prospective studies are needed in both pediatric and adult subjects to assess the generalizability of this approach of single-food elimination and are underway. Investigators in a recent multicenter study also attempted to tailor the diet using a 4-food elimination diet (milk, wheat, soy, and egg) and found a 64% response in achieving their primary endpoint of histologic remission as defined by less than 15 eos per HPF. This approach was also completed by Molina and colleagues[18] using a 4-food group elimination diet (milk, gluten-containing grains, egg, legumes) with a 54% achieved clinical histologic remission. It is hoped that future studies using empiric elimination diets will help streamline dietary therapy for patients with EoE[18] (**Table 1**).

### *Potential Development of Tolerance After Dietary Therapy*

Once a food trigger is identified in EoE, the mainstay of therapy is continued avoidance of that particular food. There have not been systematic studies looking at potential recurrent food challenges and possible development of tolerance over time. One of the first studies to address this issue was by Leung and colleagues.[19] They performed a retrospective review of EoE children who had a known diagnosis of EoE with milk as

**Table 1**
**Overview of different dietary approaches**

| | Elemental | Empirical (Most Common is SFED) | Allergy Testing–Directed |
|---|---|---|---|
| Efficacy | 91% | 72% | 41% |
| Number of Foods Avoided | All foods, pure elemental amino-acid–based formula | Typically 6, sometimes less | Can vary based on allergy testing, often <6 |
| Supporting Data | Prospective and retrospective data in pediatric and adult subjects | Prospective and retrospective data in pediatric and adult subjects | Prospective and retrospective data in pediatric and adult subject |
| Cost | $$$$ | $$ | $$ |

*Data from Refs.*[18,14]

their trigger. They identified 11 subjects who had subsequently reintroduced milk in the form of baked milk back into their diet for at least 6 weeks. Of the 15 subjects identified, 11 of them (73%) had maintained histologic remission despite reintroduction of baked milk products. The study did not mention the exact follow-up time for when reintroduction of baked milk products occurred in these subjects. Despite this limitation, this description suggests that, over time, some patients with cow's milk–induced EoE may be able to tolerate milk reintroduction in the form of baked milk, which would allow for a significant broadening of the diet.

Another study to look at this concept was performed by Dr Lucendo and colleagues[20] in adults. This group looked at the use of a cow's milk–based hydrolyzed formula in subjects with cow's milk–induced EoE. In adult subjects with cow's milk–induced EoE, 17 were administered this formula over a period of 8 weeks and repeat endoscopy was performed. At that time, 88% of subjects maintained histologic remission as defined by less than 15 eos per HPF. This study suggests that some subjects with EoE triggered by a cow's milk protein, may tolerate reintroduction of milk in this reduced antigenic state. Although these formulas are not readily accessible, this study does provide additional insight into the pathophysiologic mechanisms of food allergy triggering this disease, as well as possible tolerance to less antigenic properties of these foods.

### Potential Advantages of Dietary Therapy

Dietary therapy in adults with EoE has practical advantages. As prior studies have shown, discontinuation of swallowed topical corticosteroids in the treatment of EoE can cause symptomatic and histologic recurrence that may necessitate chronic daily therapy. Avoidance of food allergens eliminates the need for chronic medication or corticosteroids to help control the disease. Oral and esophageal candidiasis may occur in 5% to 30% of cases.[2] Other rare side effects of topical corticosteroids include growth failure in children, cataracts, and adrenal suppression. Unfortunately, these medications have not been approved by the US Food and Drug Administration to be swallowed, which raises concern about the knowledge of long-term safety with chronic use. In addition, long-term use of these medications may result in a considerable cost to patients facing this chronic condition.

The effectiveness of an elimination diet in adults supports the conceptual definition that EoE is an antigen-mediated or immune-mediated esophageal disease. Therefore, dietary therapy has the advantage of getting to the root cause of the disease; that is, food allergen avoidance, rather than symptom and histologic control with topical corticosteroids. Current consensus guidelines suggest continued avoidance of food allergens in patients who are managed with diet therapy. Therefore,[2] targeted and individualized nutrition therapy is essential to success. Recent studies have suggested that food reintroduction with altered forms of the food trigger may induce tolerance and allow for more food products to be added.

### Potential Limitations of Dietary Therapy

Although dietary therapy has advantages as previously outlined, there are practical limitations that need to be considered before suggesting this therapy for patients. One is that the foods readily available for dietary therapy are found in specialty food stores and may cost more than being on an unrestricted diet, as shown by Asher Wolf and colleagues.[21] However, the same group also has shown in a cost utility analysis of topical corticosteroids versus SFED that the topical corticosteroids are more expensive at a 5-year time horizon.[22] The major limitation of dietary therapy is the need for repeated endoscopies during the food reintroduction process to identify food triggers. The more restrictive the diet is to start, the more endoscopies are needed overall. However, there are some promising noninvasive techniques being developed to monitor esophageal inflammation.

The first technique studied was the esophageal string test, which was developed by Drs Furuta and Ackerman[23] using a string embedded in a capsule. As the capsule is swallowed, the string is deployed and maintains contact with the esophageal mucosa and adheres to fluid that contains eos byproducts. In a preliminary study, this technique showed good correlation with findings in esophageal biopsies.[23] Another technique is the use of the cytosponge device, which was initially devised to study Barrett's esophagus. This device has been used to study tissue samples from the esophagus and has also shown significant promise in correlation of eos density to that seen with standard esophageal biopsies.[24] Transnasal endoscopy has also been studied as an alternate method in both children and adults and shows good tolerability, as well as good sampling of the esophagus.[25,26] As these techniques are further refined, they may be used to assess the esophagus during food reintroduction and provide a less invasive and costly method for patients undergoing assessment in either dietary therapy or in changes with other forms of medical therapy.

Also, before advising patients on dietary therapy, it is important to have the infrastructure to be able to guide patients through this process seamlessly. Access to nutritional services and counseling for the patients is essential to help educate and monitor patients on dietary therapy, as well as provide nutritional support during this time. Resources are available and accessible to both clinicians and patients to help with this process.[27]

### SUMMARY

When discussing options for therapy with patients, it is important to review the pros and cons of each treatment plan and try to identify goals of treatment with the patient. Due to its effectiveness, dietary therapy should be offered to all EoE patients. It is important to underscore that the goals of dietary therapy are not to stay on the elemental diet or empiric elimination diets indefinitely but rather to undergo a process of food-trigger identification to help tailor the diet for long-term maintenance therapy if the diet works. The general goal of EoE therapy is to help control symptoms and histology with minimal disruption to daily routine and to maintain these goals. The choice on proceeding with medical or dietary therapy should be individualized based on patient preference, as well as available local resources.

## REFERENCES

1. Liacouras CA, Furuta GT, Hirano I, et al. Eosinophilic esophagitis: updated consensus recommendations for children and adults. J Allergy Clin Immunol 2011;128:3–20.e6 [quiz: 21–2].
2. Dellon ES, Gonsalves N, Hirano I, et al. ACG clinical guideline: evidenced based approach to the diagnosis and management of esophageal eosinophilia and eosinophilic esophagitis (EoE). Am J Gastroenterol 2013;108:679–92 [quiz: 693].
3. Kelly KJ, Lazenby AJ, Rowe PC, et al. Eosinophilic esophagitis attributed to gastroesophageal reflux: improvement with an amino acid-based formula. Gastroenterology 1995;109:1503–12.
4. Markowitz JE, Spergel JM, Ruchelli E, et al. Elemental diet is an effective treatment for eosinophilic esophagitis in children and adolescents. Am J Gastroenterol 2003;98:777–82.
5. Kagalwalla AF, Sentongo TA, Ritz S, et al. Effect of six-food elimination diet on clinical and histologic outcomes in eosinophilic esophagitis. Clin Gastroenterol Hepatol 2006;4:1097–102.
6. Kagalwalla AF, Shah A, Li BU, et al. Identification of specific foods responsible for inflammation in children with eosinophilic esophagitis successfully treated with empiric elimination diet. J Pediatr Gastroenterol Nutr 2011;53:145–9.
7. Gonsalves N, Yang GY, Doerfler B, et al. Elimination diet effectively treats eosinophilic esophagitis in adults; food reintroduction identifies causative factors. Gastroenterology 2012;142:1451–9.e1 [quiz: e14–5].
8. Liacouras CA, Spergel JM, Ruchelli E, et al. Eosinophilic esophagitis: a 10-year experience in 381 children. Clin Gastroenterol Hepatol 2005;3:1198–206.
9. Spergel JM, Brown-Whitehorn TF, Cianferoni A, et al. Identification of causative foods in children with eosinophilic esophagitis treated with an elimination diet. J Allergy Clin Immunol 2012;130:461–7.e5.
10. Lucendo AJ, Arias A, Gonzalez-Cervera J, et al. Empiric 6-food elimination diet induced and maintained prolonged remission in patients with adult eosinophilic esophagitis: a prospective study on the food cause of the disease. J Allergy Clin Immunol 2013;131:797–804.
11. Peterson KA, Byrne KR, Vinson LA, et al. Elemental diet induces histologic response in adult eosinophilic esophagitis. Am J Gastroenterol 2013;108:759–66.
12. Spergel JM, Andrews T, Brown-Whitehorn TF, et al. Treatment of eosinophilic esophagitis with specific food elimination diet directed by a combination of skin prick and patch tests. Ann Allergy Asthma Immunol 2005;95:336–43.
13. Molina-Infante J, Martin-Noguerol E, Alvarado-Arenas M, et al. Selective elimination diet based on skin testing has suboptimal efficacy for adult eosinophilic esophagitis. J Allergy Clin Immunol 2012;130:1200–2.
14. Lucendo AJ. Meta-analysis-based guidance for dietary management in eosinophilic esophagitis. Curr Gastroenterol Rep 2015;17:464.
15. Warners MJ, Vlieg-Boerstra BJ, Bredenoord AJ. Elimination and elemental diet therapy in eosinophilic oesophagitis. Best Pract Res Clin Gastroenterol 2015;29:793–803.
16. Simon D, Straumann A, Wenk A, et al. Eosinophilic esophagitis in adults–no clinical relevance of wheat and rye sensitizations. Allergy 2006;61:1480–3.

17. Kagalwalla AF, Amsden K, Shah A, et al. Cow's milk elimination: a novel dietary approach to treat eosinophilic esophagitis. J Pediatr Gastroenterol Nutr 2012; 55:711–6.
18. Molina-Infante J, Arias A, Barrio J, et al. Four-food group elimination diet for adult eosinophilic esophagitis: a prospective multicenter study. J Allergy Clin Immunol 2014;134:1093–9.e1.
19. Leung J, Hundal NV, Katz AJ, et al. Tolerance of baked milk in patients with cow's milk-mediated eosinophilic esophagitis. J Allergy Clin Immunol 2013;132: 1215–6.e1.
20. Lucendo AJ, Arias A, Gonzalez-Cervera J, et al. Tolerance of a cow's milk-based hydrolyzed formula in patients with eosinophilic esophagitis triggered by milk. Allergy 2013;68:1065–72.
21. Asher Wolf W, Huang KZ, Durban R, et al. The six-food elimination diet for eosinophilic esophagitis increases grocery shopping cost and complexity. Dysphagia 2016;31(6):765–70.
22. Cotton CC, Erim D, Eluri S, et al. Cost utility analysis of topical steroids compared with dietary elimination for treatment of eosinophilic esophagitis. Clin Gastroenterol Hepatol 2017;15:841–9.e1.
23. Furuta GT, Kagalwalla AF, Lee JJ, et al. The oesophageal string test: a novel, minimally invasive method measures mucosal inflammation in eosinophilic oesophagitis. Gut 2013;62:1395–405.
24. Katzka DA, Geno DM, Ravi A, et al. Accuracy, safety, and tolerability of tissue collection by Cytosponge vs endoscopy for evaluation of eosinophilic esophagitis. Clin Gastroenterol Hepatol 2015;13:77–83.e2.
25. Friedlander JA, DeBoer EM, Soden JS, et al. Unsedated transnasal esophagoscopy for monitoring therapy in pediatric eosinophilic esophagitis. Gastrointest Endosc 2016;83:299–306.e1.
26. Philpott H, Nandurkar S, Royce SG, et al. Ultrathin unsedated transnasal gastroscopy in monitoring eosinophilic esophagitis. J Gastroenterol Hepatol 2016;31: 590–4.
27. Doerfler B, Bryce P, Hirano I, et al. Practical approach to implementing dietary therapy in adults with eosinophilic esophagitis: the Chicago experience. Dis Esophagus 2015;28:42–58.

# Endoscopic Treatment of Eosinophilic Esophagitis

Joel E. Richter, MD, MACG

## KEYWORDS

- Esophageal dilation • Maloney and Savary bougies • Through-the-scope balloons
- Esophageal perforation • Chest pain • Deep tears • Eosinophilic esophagitis
- Strictures

## KEY POINTS

- Tissue remodeling with fibrosis is the main cause of solid-food dysphagia and food impactions in adult patients with eosinophilic esophagitis (EoE).
- Simple endoscopy is not accurate for determining the degree and location of strictures; careful bougie dilation can be more helpful.
- Gradual bougie/balloon dilation to 17 to 18 mm is safe and can relieve dysphagia symptoms for an average of 2 years.
- Slow and gradual dilation is the key to success. Some postdilation chest pain is expected.
- Some healthy adult patients with EoE prefer an occasional esophageal dilation to regular use of medications or restricted diet.

## INTRODUCTION

Eosinophilic esophagitis (EoE) was first recognized as an inflammatory disease of the esophagus with mucosal eosinophilia, but over the last 10 years it has been slowly recognized that esophageal remodeling with stricture disease is an important feature of this disease in adult, and sometimes adolescent, patients. Historically and in early guidelines,[1] endoscopic treatment with esophageal dilation was relegated to a small number of patients with intractable strictures and was thought to be dangerous with a high rate of chest pain and perforations. Esophageal dilation, especially for patients with the fibrostenotic phenotype of EoE, is now a highly effective, immediate, and safe therapy for relieving dysphagia that can provide long-term relief of dysphagia with or without concomitant medical or dietary therapy.

Conflicts of Interest: The author has no commercial or financial conflicts of interest.
Division of Digestive Diseases & Nutrition, Joy McCann Culverhouse Center for Swallowing Disorders, University of South Florida Morsani College of Medicine, 12901 Bruce B. Downs Boulevard, MDC 72, Tampa, FL 33612, USA
E-mail address: Jrichte1@health.usf.edu

## CLINICAL ASSESSMENT OF ESOPHAGEAL REMODELING

In children, EoE is more of an inflammatory process with symptoms of failure to thrive, vomiting, heartburn, and abdominal pain. In adolescents and adults, the symptoms are primarily solid-food dysphagia, heartburn, and chest pain that can be associated with food impactions with or without strictures.[1] Esophageal strictures are present in 30% to 80% of adults with EoE, but are less frequent in children (5%–10%), although approximately one-third experience food impactions. Two studies from Switzerland and the United States[2,3] confirm that the presence and severity of stricture disease coincide with a longer duration of undiagnosed disease. These changes in clinical features are the results of disease evolution from a predominately inflammatory process, which, if left untreated for many years, results in esophageal remodeling with fibrosis, rings, strictures, and generalized esophageal narrowing.[4]

### History

The symptom of dysphagia for solid foods in patients with EoE is a complex pathophysiologic process with both mechanical and psychological factors. Although the inciting event is the mucosal eosinophilic inflammation, the degree of mucosal eosinophilia does not correlate with the severity of dysphagia.[5] As shown in **Fig. 1**, dysphagia is related to mechanical factors that include the degree of dysmotility present, and the extent of mucosal inflammation and fibrostenosis from esophageal remodeling.[6] The contribution of each may vary in individual patients and be incompletely evaluated by endoscopy with biopsies alone. Furthermore, treatments tend to address only 1 of these mechanisms. Thus, patients on topical steroids or dietary therapy might continue to experience dysphagia despite adequate antiinflammatory medications, if fibrostenosis or severe dysmotility is not recognized.

### Barium Esophagram

The barium esophagram is a cheap and readily available test to assess esophageal remodeling and identify areas with strictures. Before the term EoE, radiograph patterns in these patients were associated with several aliases for this disease, including

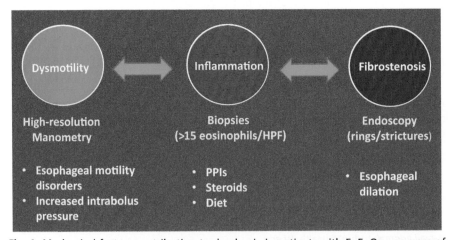

**Fig. 1.** Mechanical factors contributing to dysphagia in patients with EoE. One or more of these factors may contribute to symptoms and food impactions. HPF, high-power field; PPIs, proton pump inhibitors. (*From* Richter JE. New guidelines for eosinophilic esophagitis. Will it measure what we want? Gastroenterology 2014;147:1212–3; with permission.)

ringed esophagus, corrugated esophagus, feline esophagus, small-caliber or narrowed esophagus, and congenital esophageal stenosis.[7–11] A recent study from the Mayo Clinic[12] confirms that the barium esophagram is the most accurate test for identifying esophageal narrowing and multiple strictures. Among healthy subjects in the upright position, the maximal esophageal diameter while continuously drinking barium was greater than 21 mm and the minimal diameter between swallows was greater than 16 mm.[12] Using this technique in 58 patients with EoE also undergoing endoscopy, endoscopy had poor sensitivity (14.7%) and only modest specificity (79.2%) for identifying esophageal strictures. Even at a cutoff diameter of less than 15 mm, endoscopy only had a sensitivity of 25% for a narrowed esophagus.

## Endoscopy

In practice, upper endoscopy is the first test done in patients with suspected EoE to inspect the esophagus, obtain biopsies, identify strictures, treat food impactions, and exclude alternative diagnoses (**Fig. 2**A, B). However, even using the new Endoscopic Reference Scoring System (EREFS),[13] the diagnostic reliability of endoscopy is variable, especially for esophageal remodeling: interobserver agreement for rings, furrows, and exudate was moderate (56%–65% agreement); fair for narrowed-caliber esophagus; and poor for edema and feline esophagus. Furthermore, the system is crude for defining the degree of esophageal lumen narrowing. Strictures are scored as grade 0 (absent) and grade 1 (present). Fixed rings are graded as 0, none; 1, mild and subtle; 2, moderate (does not impair passage of an adult endoscope; 8–9.5 mm); and 3, severe (distinct rings that do not permit passage of the adult endoscope).[13]

Because the ability of endoscopy to identify strictures is unreliable, we found that a simple assessment of bougie size, at the time of initial endoscopy, is better than visual inspection alone and easy to perform. After biopsies are obtained, we routinely dilate all patients with EoE to assess lumen diameter, defined by the bougie size at which moderate resistance is noted with the passage of Savary or Maloney dilators. We find that one-third of our patients with EoE have subtle strictures, sometimes multiple, between 10 and 17 mm, that may not reliably be detected with endoscopy alone.[3]

## Other Tests: Manometry and Functional Luminal Imaging Probe Technology

Esophageal manometry commonly finds nonspecific esophageal motility patterns or low lower esophageal sphincter pressure in patients with EoE. High-resolution manometry has identified a novel finding in patients with EoE, probably related to esophageal fibrosis and poor distensibility, characterized by distal esophageal

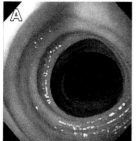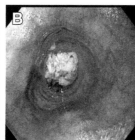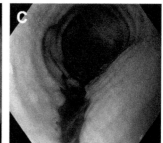

**Fig. 2.** (*A*) Classic EoE with multiple rings. (*B*) Fibrostenotic EoE with rings and food impaction. (*C*) Esophageal mucosal tear after dilation in a patient with EoE.

pressurization (measured by intrabolus pressure) in 34% to 48% of adult patients with EoE.[14,15] We have confirmed these findings in 29 patients with EoE, observing that the average intrabolus pressure was significantly higher (P<.05) in fibrostenotic versus inflammatory EoE (18.6 vs 12.6 mm).[16] A dramatic example of this is shown in **Fig. 3**, in which the fibrosis essentially trapped the esophageal body, preventing normal peristalsis and bolus clearance. Esophageal dilation from 8 mm to 17 mm, without improvement in mucosal eosinophilia, resolved the patient's dysphagia and her esophageal motility returned to normal.

Functional luminal imaging probe (FLIP) is a novel system that can be used at endoscopy to measure the distensibility of the esophageal wall. Studies have shown that 50% of patients with EoE have reduced esophageal distensibility compared with controls[17] and that those patients with EoE with a history of food impaction had lower distensibility parameters than those with solid-food dysphagia alone.[18] A recent study using FLIP technology validated the EREFS scoring system for rings, finding that higher ring scores[2,3] were associated with lower distensibility (r = −0.46; P<.0001). The severity of exudates and furrows and the degree of mucosal eosinophilia did not correlate with distensibility parameters.[19]

### Personal historical perspective on the role of esophageal dilation in eosinophilic esophagitis

My personal experience of EoE is presented here, based on my 35 years as an esophagologist. In previous writings, I compared this experience with medieval history, with the Dark Ages and then the Renaissance.[20,21] In preparing this article, I also see some similarities to the parable of the blind men describing the elephant.

In retrospect, I saw my first case of probable EoE in the early 1980s when a young white man from North Carolina presented to the hospital with a food impaction.

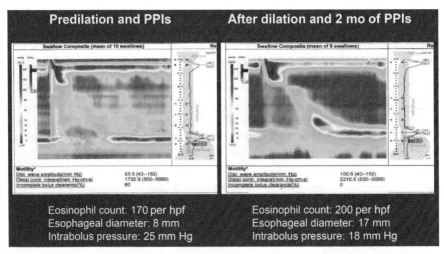

**Fig. 3.** Predilation and postdilation high-resolution esophageal manometry in a young woman with EoE and narrowed esophagus. Initial manometry found weak peristalsis with impaired bolus clearance (60%) and high intrabolus pressure. After 5 sessions of gradual esophageal dilation from 8 mm to 17 mm, distal wave amplitude and distal contractile integral has increased, esophageal bolus clearance is normal, and intrabolus pressure has decreased to near normal. However, the inflammatory process was unchanged after 2 months of twice-daily PPI therapy. This finding suggests that the fibrotic scarring was trapping the esophageal body, preventing normal peristalsis and clearance.

Endoscopy showed striking rings, but biopsies were not done. He improved with esophageal dilation and $H_2$ antagonists. Several other cases were seen over the next 10 years. I was intrigued by Attwood and colleagues'[22] report in 1993 of 12 patients with dysphagia and marked mucosal eosinophilia without evidence of gastroesophageal reflux disease (GERD). However, they observed that endoscopy was normal in their patients, unlike my few cases with multiple rings.

My group published our first article on the ringed esophagus at the Cleveland Clinic in 2001. This article described 19 patients treated over the previous 4 years with demographic features of EoE, solid-food dysphagia, and history of food impactions.[7] All had many eosinophils on their esophageal biopsies but also basal cell hyperplasia and prolongation of the rete pegs. Therefore, my gastrointestinal pathologist, John Goldblum, interpreted these features as GERD, as was the pathology teaching at the time.[23] All patients improved with esophageal dilations to 14 to 15 mm and proton pump inhibitors (PPIs). Different from routine peptic strictures, pain with deep tears was common after these dilations. Telephone follow-up in 16 patients found that all were doing well with occasional dysphagia after an average of 19 months posttreatment. One patient failed 3 dilation sessions and did well on oral prednisone per the Attwood and colleagues[22] experience. Two years later, in their first report in the English literature, Straumann and colleagues[24] from Switzerland reported on 11 adult patients with a new syndrome of primary EoE who were treated with esophageal dilation alone. Dilation was successful in 10 patients, with symptom relief from 1 to 24 months. The investigators also noted "impressive lacerations"[24] after the dilations, but these were well tolerated by the patients.

Soon thereafter, case reports began to highlight high rates of mucosal tears, chest pain, and need for hospitalization, and there were rare reports of esophageal perforation. In total, 84 adult patients with EoE reported before 2008 underwent esophageal dilation, with 5% experiencing esophageal perforations and 7% requiring hospitalization; a rate that was much higher than for peptic esophageal strictures.[25]

During these Dark Ages, I was invited to the First International Gastrointestinal Eosinophil Research Symposium in Orlando (October 17–18, 2006), sponsored by the North American Society for Pediatric Gastroenterology, Hepatology and Nutrition. The audience was mostly pediatric gastroenterologists, allergists, pathologists, and basic scientists, and only a few adult esophagologists (H. Worth Boyce, Stuart Spechler, David Katzka, Ikuo Hirano, Amindra Arora). Like the analogy of the blind men and the elephant, it soon became obvious that our colleagues were describing a different esophageal disease than we were treating, characterized by an allergic inflammatory response responding to topical steroids or food elimination diets. Appeals went out to stop dilating these patients with EoE because it was dangerous and harmful. Following this meeting, the first international EoE guidelines were published in 2007 and recommended that, "whenever possible medical or dietary therapy should be attempted prior to performing esophageal dilation."[1] However, myself and other experienced adult esophagologists continued to safely dilate our patients with EoE as primary treatment while developing thriving referral practices from community physicians fearful of esophageal dilation and patients seeking symptom relief after failing medical therapies.

The following 3 to 4 years were interesting because I lectured across the country and vigorously debated the role of esophageal dilation in EoE. Fortunately, 2010 heralded the Renaissance period with the publication of 3 articles (1 from my group at Temple) detailing our success treating patients with EoE with strictures using both bougies and through-the-scope (TTS) balloons.[26–28] In a total of 109 adults, the results were remarkably consistent: patients were easily dilated over 1 to 3 sessions to esophageal diameters of 16 to 17 mm with 91% of patients experiencing dysphagia relief for an average of 22 to 24 months. Mucosal eosinophilia did not change and complications were infrequent: 3 tears and no perforations. Subsequently, there have been nearly 1000 patients with EoE reported in the world literature who were treated safely with similar efficacy using careful techniques of esophageal dilation. With much pleasure, I actively participated on the second international EoE guidelines in 2011, which began to liberalize their recommendations: "Esophageal dilation with or without concomitant medical or dietary therapy can provide relief of dysphagia in selected cases. In the absence of high grade esophageal stenosis, a trial of medical or dietary therapy before esophageal dilation is reasonable. For high grade strictures, dilation before initiation of medical therapy has been well tolerated and effective."[5] This recommendation represented a vindication of esophageal dilation.

### General efficacy of esophageal dilation for eosinophilic esophagitis

A recent meta-analysis reviewed the clinical efficacy of esophageal dilation for the treatment of EoE. Moawad and colleagues[29] identified 27 studies meeting inclusion criteria. Overall, there were 2873 patients with EoE, of whom 1112 were children (<18 years). The mean age was 32.5 years, 75% were men, and 100% experienced dysphagia, with 59% reporting food impactions. Rings were the most common endoscopic feature, reported in 73% of patients. The most common medical therapies used were topical steroids (58%), PPIs (56%), and diet (12%). Among the studies, 845 patients with EoE (29.4%) underwent a total of 1820 esophageal dilations, with a mean of 2 sessions per patient and a range from 1 to 35 dilations per patient. The method of dilation included 149 Maloney, 433 Savary, and 759 TTS balloons. Among the 8 studies reporting esophageal diameter before and after dilation, the mean predilation lumen was 9.9 mm and the mean postdilation diameter was 16.1 mm. Most of the strictures were in the distal esophagus (73.6%). Clinical improvement from dilation occurred in 95% of patients with EoE following dilation (95% confidence interval, 90%–98%). The duration of improvement was reported in 13 studies and ranged from a median of 1 week to 36 weeks. Complications were rare.

This group did a similar meta-analysis on the available adult literature published before 2013.[30] Since then the number of reported patients undergoing dilation has more than doubled and there has been a 3-fold increase in the number of endoscopic procedures. Compared with their earlier study, the effectiveness has increased by 15% and, importantly, heterogeneity in clinical improvement has decreased from 86% to 10%, suggesting the highly consistent reliability of esophageal dilation among studies published over the last 3 years.

### Safety of esophageal dilation in patients with eosinophilic esophagitis

Two large recent meta-analyses evaluated the safety of esophageal dilation for patients with EoE. The first study was by Moawad and colleagues[29] (discussed previously) and the second was by Dougherty and colleagues.[31] Although performed around the same time, the latter study recorded a larger group of 32 studies,[32] including 977 patients representing 2034 esophageal dilations. Nevertheless, as summarized in **Table 1**, the safety of esophageal dilation in patients with EoE is indisputable, perforations are rare, and there have been no deaths.

The deep esophageal tears and fear about perforations encountered during endoscopic treatments are not surprising because of the marked fibrosis-driven esophageal fragility (so-called crepe paper esophagus) of EoE. We observed in a recent review,[33] esophageal perforations can occur from multiple factors, including severe

| Table 1 | | | | | | | |
|---|---|---|---|---|---|---|---|
| Summary of the reported world experience with complications from esophageal dilation in patients with eosinophilic esophagitis | | | | | | | |
| | Total EoE | | Complications per Dilation | | | | |
| Study | Patients Dilated (N) | Dilations (N) | Hospitalizations (%) | Perforations (%) | Hemorrhage (%) | Chest Pain (%) | Death |
| Moawad et al,[29] 2017 | 845 | 1820 | 0.67 | 0.38 | 0.05 | 9.3 | 0 |
| Dougherty et al,[31] 2017 | 977 | 2034 | 0.69 | 0.03 | 0.03 | 3.6 | 0 |

retching with Boerhaave syndrome; passage of rigid instruments by ear, nose, and throat physicians; passage of a flexible endoscope alone; and esophageal dilation. The Dougherty and colleagues[31] meta-analysis identified a total of 9 perforations with a perforation rate of 0.03% per procedure. Data were available on 6 cases, with 5 being designated as so-called contained perforations (computed tomography scan showing extraluminal air only). Only 1 was transmural with Gastrografin extravasation and pooling in the pleural space.[34] All 6 perforations were treated medically and no deaths occurred. The investigators also observed that most perforations (5 out of 9) were from publications before 2009. The perforation rate for cases reported before 2009 was 0.41% (5 out of 203 procedures) and dramatically decreased from 2009 onward to 0.03% (4 out of 1831 procedures). These differences may be caused by publication bias in the early smaller series, but more likely gastroenterologists are more aware of EoE and are adapting better dilation techniques to maximize the safety of the procedure. Perforation rates in the 30 studies with details of dilator preferences found no difference between bougies (0.02%; 2 out of 1120 procedures) and balloon dilators (0.06%; 2 out of 837 procedures). Therefore, the perforation rate in EoE-related strictures is similar to the 0.4% cited for other benign causes of esophageal strictures,[35] and lower than that of refractory strictures.[36]

In contrast, mucosal tears associated with some degree of chest pain are common after dilating patients with EoE (see **Fig. 2**C). In my experience, chest pain after dilating patients with EoE is nearly universal but is only reported in 5% to 10% of studies, with a wide range from 0.63% to 100%.[29] Some of this variation is related to the definition (minimal mucosal disruption to deep mucosal tears) or technique used for dilation (ie, TTS balloons allow easier assessment of tears). These tears are not true complications but are an indicator of effective esophageal dilation in which the goal is to disrupt the collagen-rich tissue. However, some of this is reporting bias, as shown by the Schoepfer and colleagues[26] study, in which chest pain was self-reported in 74% of patients and usually considered mild, but was noted in only 7% of the medical records. Some patients require narcotic analgesia, but most easily respond to reassurance and nonsteroidal antiinflammatory drugs (NSAIDs). Deep tears requiring hospitalization do not require surgery and respond to conservative therapy, usually over 1 to 5 days.

Several reports have attempted to identify risk factors for esophageal complications. Most are consistent with the concept that severe remodeling with scar tissue results in a more fragile esophageal wall. These factors include strictures in the proximal and midesophagus, tight strictures, long duration, and high eosinophil count.[28,32,34] The recent Dougherty and colleagues[31] meta-analysis only found that esophageal perforations were more common with larger dilators (>17 mm) than smaller dilators and rates were lower in pediatric compared with adult studies.

### Guidelines for safe esophageal dilation

Only recently have there been recommendations from GI societies about esophageal dilation in patients with EoE.[37] The key for all gastroenterologists is to follow the simple tenet to start low and go slow when dilating these patients. These dilations are not like the treatment of peptic strictures or rings, for which big is better, pain is uncommon, and the important narrowing is always at the esophagogastric junction.

I prefer bougie dilations, as summarized in **Box 1**.[38,39] All patients must be forewarned of pain, which may persist for 1 to 7 days. I find that this recognition reduces patients' fears, results in fewer telephone calls, and helps them tolerate the pain using mild analgesics. Because the esophagus may be narrowed in multiple sites or diffusely in up to 25% of patients, my dilators of choice are the Savary-Guillard or Maloney bougies, which reliably dilate the entire length of the esophagus and give better tactile assessment of the location and degree of esophageal narrowing. Strictures less than 15 mm are usually dilated with Savary bougies over a guidewire and then I switch to Maloney bougies for larger diameters. I rarely need fluoroscopy but always have available a transnasal 5-mm endoscope for the very tight strictures. Dilations are started with small-diameter bougies and progressed at the first setting until a diameter of 17 mm is easily obtained or moderate resistance with or without blood is noted. The rule of 3 is not followed but perhaps should be for endoscopists less experienced with dilation. All patients are dilated during the first endoscopy session after biopsies are obtained regardless of whether they are receiving any medical therapy. I believe this is the most reliable means to separate the inflammatory from the fibrostenotic features of EoE. In addition, I do not look for tears because I know from experience and my tactile sensation that they will be present when moderate resistance to the bougie's passage is encountered (see **Fig. 2**C). Other investigators[38] routinely inspect

---

**Box 1**
**General guidelines for esophageal dilation in patients with eosinophilic esophagitis**

- Forewarn the patient that some degree of pain postdilation is to be expected and that it will respond to NSAIDs.

- Examine the entire esophagus before dilation to assess the location of strictures and estimate esophageal diameter. Have available a pediatric or 5-mm transnasal endoscope for tight strictures, minimizing the need for fluoroscopy and blind dilations.

- Start low, with small-diameter bougies/balloons and gradually dilate to 16 to 18 mm. May require several sessions separated by 3 to 4 weeks.

- Limit the progression of dilation per session to moderate resistance to bougie passage, blood on the dilator, or significant tears.

- Look for tears if you must, but they only represent an adequate dilation.

- After induction dilation sessions to 16 to 18 mm, repeat dilations are triggered by recurrence of dysphagia complaints. Many patients only need maintenance dilations every 2 to 3 years.

- Dilation therapy should usually be done in conjunction with medical treatment (PPIs, steroids, diet) to reduce the rate of stricture recurrence by treating the underlying inflammation.

*Modified from* Richter JE. Eosinophilic esophagitis dilation in the community – try it – you will like it – but start low and go slow. Am J Gastroenterol 2016;111:215; with permission.

the esophageal mucosa after dilation increments of 1 to 2 mm or after encountering resistance to bougie passage. I think the latter approach is helpful for physicians who do not do frequent dilations and are uncomfortable estimating the resistance tolerated for esophageal dilation. My technique of bougie dilation only adds 1 to 2 minutes to the procedure and the bougies are reusable.

My goal in dilating patients with EoE is to start with a smaller diameter bougie, progress slowly with dilation sessions every 3 to 4 weeks, and get all patients to a minimum bougie diameter of 16 to 18 mm. This degree of lumen diameter allows patients to eat a modified regular diet (15 mm, 45 French) or a full regular diet (18 mm, 54 French).[40] For minimal strictures, this can be done in the initial diagnostic session, whereas tight strictures may require on average 2 to 5 sessions (10 is my record) while they also receive medical therapy (usually PPIs as part of a trial). This induction phase rapidly relieves their dysphagia independently of medical therapy, most patients can eat a regular diet, and food impactions are eliminated. After completion, it is critical to place these patients with fibrostenotic EoE into a maintenance program. Some require dilation at regular intervals (every 6 or 12 months), but I prefer to redilate only when dysphagia begins to recur at a frequency of approximately once a week. With this approach, my colleagues and I found that many patients require dilation only every 2 to 3 years, with up to nearly 20 years of follow-up.[41] This finding is compatible with our recent observation on esophageal remodeling that patients dilated to a diameter of 17 mm with bougies decrease their lumen size by $0.64 \pm 0.13$ mm/y.[42]

The University of North Carolina group primarily uses TTS balloons,[28,43] pointing to 2 theoretic advantages: radial rather than shearing forces are applied during the procedure, reducing the chance of perforation, and clinicians can immediately assess the degree of esophageal tearing. Briefly, after examining the esophagus, a multisize balloon (8, 9, 10 mm; CRE Fixed Wire Balloon Dilator, Boston Scientific) is positioned across the esophagogastric junction, if there is resistance to passage of an adult endoscope; or a 10-mm, 11-mm, 12-mm balloon if the endoscope passes easily. The balloon is inflated to the smallest diameter and, with the balloon positioned in front of the endoscope, slowly withdrawn (2–3 cm/s) from distal to proximal until the entire esophagus is examined. Lumen narrowing is appreciated by an inability to easily pull the balloon through the region. If no resistance is detected, then the procedure is repeated with the next size of balloons in serial fashion, looking for subtle tears as the balloon is withdrawn. When resistance is encountered, the balloon is deflated, repositioned across the region of resistance, and slowly reinflated until it easily passes or a tear is seen.[43] I have not tried this technique but it seems tedious and time consuming, without providing a clear understanding of how well the entire esophagus is dilated. The balloons are expensive ($150 per balloon) and not reusable. Nevertheless, their results in 164 patients are comparable with bougie series,[43] emphasizing that bougies and balloons are equally successful when used by skilled endoscopists.

## SPECIAL SITUATIONS
### Pediatric Patients

Esophageal strictures occur in only 5% to 10% of children with EoE, most of whom are adolescents.[1] The reports describing outcomes of esophageal dilations are limited.[44,45] The Denver group recently published their 5-year experience in 40 patients with EoE undergoing 68 esophageal dilations, representing approximately 5% of their EoE clinic.[45] These children were older (average 14 years old) with the diagnosis of strictures made equally with barium esophagram or endoscopy. Dilation techniques were similar to those in adults, with 72% of children being dilated with Maloney bougies, usually to a goal diameter of 15 mm. Twenty-three children (58%) had a single dilation and the remaining 17 underwent from 2 to 5 dilations with sessions separated on average by nearly 9 months. Symptoms improved in 86% of the group and complications were infrequent (2.9%) and similar to the 3.1% rate in non-EoE pediatric esophageal cases, including caustic ingestion, epidermolysis bullosa, esophageal atresia, and tracheoesophageal fistula. Two children were hospitalized overnight with chest pain but no perforations occurred.

### Patients with Previous Postdilation Complications

A rare group, patients with EoE who have deep tears with severe pain or perforation requiring hospitalization, can be problematic because after recovery most need further dilations or live a life of marked food restriction. We recently reviewed our experience with 8 of these patients referred to my practice at the University of South Florida.[46] Five had esophageal perforations, 1 required surgery, and the others had deep tears with severe pain. They were hospitalized from 1 to 17 days. Most complications occurred during the first dilation (6 out of 8; 75%) with bougie sizes from 12 to 18 mm. Esophageal dilation parameters and success were compared with 22 other patients with fibrostenotic EoE treated over the same 5 years, and these are summarized in **Table 2**. Not surprisingly, the esophageal diameter at initial dilation was smaller in the patients with prior complications; however, the end diameter was similar across both groups. The total number of sessions, as well as sessions to reach the diameter of 17 mm, were higher in the complicated patients. On average, this group took about 3.5 months to be adequately dilated, but by starting low and going slow no further complications occurred and all are doing well with follow-up of more than 1 year.

### Primary Therapy for Eosinophilic Esophagitis

The safety and durability of esophageal dilation warrants consideration for solo primary therapy for selected patients with EoE.[20] This approach is more agreeable than dietary therapy and much more reliable than steroid therapy in adults. In otherwise healthy and active young adults, I have found that 10% to 20% prefer an occasional dilation to regular use of medications or complicated diets. However, dilations as monotherapy do not treat the underlying inflammation.[26,27] I treat all my patients initially with PPIs and am satisfied with this medication alone even if patients still have mild persistent mucosal eosinophilia in the range of 15 to 40 eosinophils per high powered field. This approach is supported by our experience in a selected group

**Table 2**
**Esophageal dilation of patients with eosinophilic esophagitis with prior complications versus control group**

|  | Prior Complications: 8 Patients | No Complications: 22 Patients | P Value |
|---|---|---|---|
| Initial Diameter (mm) | 9.0 ± 1.51 (SD) | 11.73 ± 2.98 | P = .003 |
| End Diameter (mm) | 15.75 ± 1.83 | 16.09 ± 1.97 | P = .67 |
| Dilation Sessions (N) | 4.00 ± 1.77 | 2.32 ± 1.04 | P = .019 |
| Achieved 17 mm Diameter, N (%) | 4 out of 8 (50%) | 15 out of 22 (68%) | P = .37 |
| Dilation Sessions to Reach 17 mm (N) | 3.75 ± 0.96 | 2.27 ± 0.96 | P = .05 |
| Time to Reach 17 mm (mo) | 3.50 ± 0.58 | 2.33 ± 2.29 | P = .09 |
| Symptom Resolution (N) | 8 out of 8 | 22 out of 22 | — |
| Complications (N) | 0 out of 8 | 0 out of 22 | — |

of patients with EoE treated only with PPIs and serial esophageal dilation who have done well with no complications over 14 years of follow-up. On average, these patients required esophageal dilation every other year on their maintenance programs.[41] However, when the mucosal eosinophilia is greater, I treat with either topical steroids or an elimination diet based on allergy testing. It is hoped that, by further reducing the inflammation, fewer dilations will be required.

## SUMMARY

In many adults with EoE, the main cause of solid-food dysphagia is tissue remodeling resulting in strictures and narrowed esophagus. A long period of time before diagnosis associated with a more severe stricture suggests an evolution from pure inflammation to fibrosis. Endoscopy and biopsies are excellent for assessing inflammation but markedly underestimate the degree of fibrostenosis in many patients with EoE. Therefore, as shown in **Fig. 4**, a key component of my algorithm for diagnosing and treating EoE is to evaluate and treat both potential features of the disease simultaneously. My approach to the inflammatory component is similar to others, but I deviate from the guidelines by performing bougie dilation in all my patients at the initial endoscopy. If the esophagus can easily be dilated to 17 mm with minimal to no resistance, then I am confident the inflammatory phenotype dominates, medical therapy is my primary treatment, and further dilations are rarely needed. In contrast, inability to easily dilate the esophagus, even if no strictures are appreciated endoscopically, confirms the fibrostenotic phenotype and requires treatment with serial dilations over multiple sessions to a 17-mm to 18-mm lumen diameter in parallel with medical antiinflammatory therapy. The latter phenotype often needs maintenance dilations, which I perform based on symptom recurrence.

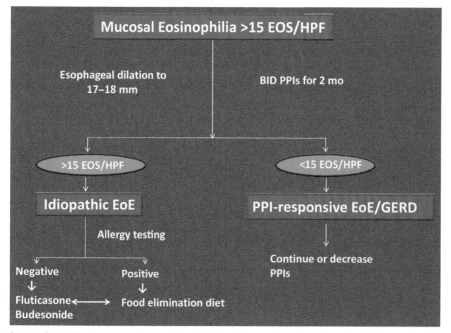

**Fig. 4.** The author's personal algorithm for the diagnosis and treatment of EoE. See text for details. BID, twice a day; EOS, eosinophils.

As the review has emphasized, esophageal dilation is no longer a barbaric, dangerous, Dark Ages treatment of EoE but is now part of the Renaissance era, in which there are 3 highly effective treatments that alleviate troublesome symptoms, allow patients to live normal lives without fear of food impactions, and prevent disease progression. Esophageal dilation is effective, safe, and easy to perform as long as clinicians remember the tenet start low and go slow. All physicians managing patients with EoE should join the enlightened age of EoE therapy, in which medical therapy and esophageal dilation are equal treatments in the treatment of these patients. Using the techniques outlined, esophageal dilation can be done as safely in the community setting as in the academic centers. Try it; you will like it and your patients will get immediate and long-term benefit.

## REFERENCES

1. Furuta GT, Liacouras CA, Collins MH, et al. Eosinophilic esophagitis in children and adults: a systematic review and consensus recommendation for diagnosis and treatment. Gastroenterology 2007;133:1342–63.
2. Schoepfer AM, Safroneeva E, Bussman C, et al. Delay in diagnosis of eosinophilia esophagitis increases risk of stricture formation in a time-dependent manner. Gastroenterology 2013;145:1230–6.
3. Lipka S, Kumar A, Richter JE. Impact of diagnostic delay and other risk factors on eosinophilic esophagitis phenotype and esophageal diameter. J Clin Gastroenterol 2016;50:134–40.
4. Hirano I, Aceves SS. Clinical implications and pathogenesis of esophageal remodeling in eosinophilic esophagitis. Gastroenterol Clin North Am 2014;43:297–311.
5. Liacouras CA, Furuta GT, Hirano I, et al. Eosinophilic esophagitis: updated consensus recommendations for children and adults. J Allergy Clin Immunol 2011;129:3–20.
6. Richter JE. New guidelines for eosinophilic esophagitis. Will it measure what we want? Gastroenterology 2014;147:1212–3.
7. Morrow JB, Vargo JJ, Goldblum JR, et al. The ringed esophagus: features of GERD. Am J Gastroenterol 2001;96:984–9.
8. Langdon DE. Corrugated ringed esophagus. Am J Gastroenterol 1993;88:1461.
9. Potter JW, Saeian K, Staff D, et al. Eosinophilic esophagitis in adults: an emerging problem with unique esophageal features. Gastrointest Endosc 2004;59:355–61.
10. Renker IO, Hemar MB, Peu HA, et al. Ringed esophagus (feline esophagus) in childhood. Pediatr Radiol 1997;27:773–5.
11. Langdon DE. Congenital esophageal stenosis, corrugated esophagus and eosinophilic esophagitis. Am J Gastroenterol 2000;95:2123–4.
12. Gentile N, Katzka D, Ravi K, et al. Oesophageal narrowing is common and frequently under- appreciated at endoscopy in patients with oesophageal eosinophilia. Aliment Pharmacol Ther 2014;40:1333–40.
13. Hirano I, Moy N, Heckman MG, et al. Endoscopic assessment of the oesophageal features of eosinophilic oesophagitis: validation of a novel classification system. Gut 2013;62:489–95.
14. Roman S, Hirano I, Kwiatek MA, et al. Manometric features of eosinophilic esophagitis in esophageal pressure topography. Neurogastroenterol Motil 2011;23:208–14.

15. Martin L, Santander C, Lopez Martin MC, et al. Esophageal motor abnormalities in eosinophilic esophagitis identified by high resolution manometry. J Gastroenterol Hepatol 2011;26:1447–56.

16. Colizzo JM, Clayton SB, Richter JE. Intrabolus pressure on high resolution manometry distinguishes fibrostenotic and inflammatory phenotypes of EoE. Dig Esophagus 2016;29:551–7.

17. Kwiatek MA, Hirano I, Kahrilas PJ, et al. Mechanical properties of the esophagus in eosinophilic esophagitis. Gastroenterology 2011;140:82–90.

18. Nicodeme F, Hirano I, Chen J, et al. Eosinophilic distensibility as a measure of disease severity in patients with eosinophilic esophagitis. Clin Gastroenterol Hepatol 2013;11:1101–7.

19. Chen JW, Pandolfino JF, Lin Z, et al. Severity of endoscopically identified esophageal rings correlates with reduced esophageal distensibility in eosinophilic esophagitis. Endoscopy 2016;48:794–801.

20. Richter JE. Esophageal dilation in eosinophilic esophagitis. Best Pract Res Clin Gastroenterol 2015;29:815–28.

21. Richter JE. Current management of eosinophilic esophagitis 2015. J Clin Gastroenterol 2016;2:99–110.

22. Attwood SEA, Smyrk TR, DeMeester TR, et al. Esophageal eosinophilia with dysphagia. A distinct clinicopathologic syndrome. Dig Dis Sci 1993;38:109–16.

23. Winters HS, Madara JL, Stafford RJ, et al. Intraepithelial eosinophils: a new diagnostic criterion for reflux esophagitis. Gastroenterology 1982;83:818–23.

24. Straumann A, Spichtin HP, Grize L, et al. Natural history of primary eosinophilic esophagitis: a follow-up of 30 adult patients for up to 11.5 years. Gastroenterology 2003;125:1660–9.

25. Hirano I. Dilation in eosinophilic esophagitis: to do or not to do. Gastrointest Endosc 2010;71(4):713–4.

26. Schoepfer AM, Gonsalves N, Bassman C, et al. Esophageal dilation in eosinophilic esophagitis: effectiveness, safety and impact on underlying inflammation. Am J Gastroenterol 2010;105:1062–70.

27. Bohm M, Richter JE, Kelsen S, et al. Esophageal dilation: simple and effective treatment for adults with eosinophilic esophagitis and esophageal rings and strictures. Dis Esophagus 2010;23:377–85.

28. Dellon ES, Gibbs WB, Rubinas TC, et al. Esophageal dilation in eosinophilic esophagitis: safety and predictors of clinical response and complications. Gastrointest Endosc 2010;71:706–12.

29. Moawad F, Molina-Infante J, Lucendo A, et al. Endoscopic dilation is highly effective and safe in children and adults with eosinophilic esophagitis: a systematic review and meta-analysis. Aliment Pharmacol Ther 2017;46(2):96–105.

30. Moawad F, Cheatham JG, DeZee KJ. Meta-analysis: the safety and efficacy of dilation in eosinophilic oesophagitis. Aliment Pharmacol Ther 2013;38:713–20.

31. Dougherty M, Runge TM, Eluri S, et al. Esophageal dilation with either bougie or balloon technique is a safe treatment for eosinophilic esophagitis: a systematic review and meta- analysis. Gastrointest Endosc 2017;86(4):581–91.

32. Cohen MS, Kaufman AB, Palazzo JP, et al. An audit of endoscopic complications in adult eosinophilic esophagitis. Clin Gastroenterol Hepatol 2007;5(10):1149–53.

33. Bohm ME, Richter JE. Review article: oesophageal dilation in adults with eosinophilic esophagitis. Aliment Pharmacol Ther 2011;37:748–57.

34. Jung KW, Gundersen N, Kopacova J, et al. Occurrence of and risk factors for complications after endoscopic dilation in eosinophilic esophagitis. Gastrointest Endosc 2011;73:15–21.

35. Siersema PD, de Wijkerslooth LRH. Dilation of refractory benign esophageal strictures. Gastrointest Endosc 2009;70:1000–12.
36. Repici A, Small AJ, Mendleson A, et al. Natural history and management of refractory benign esophageal strictures. Gastrointest Endosc 2016;84:222–8.
37. Dellon ES, Gonsalves N, Hirano I, et al. ACG guideline: evidence based approach to the diagnosis and management of esophageal eosinophilia and eosinophilic esophagitis. Am J Gastroenterol 2013;108:679–92.
38. Richter JE. Eosinophilic esophagitis dilation in the community – try it – you will like it – but start low and go slow. Am J Gastroenterol 2016;111:214–6.
39. Hirano I. How I approach the management of eosinophilic esophagitis in adults. Am J Gastroenterol 2017;112:197–9.
40. Goldschmid S, Boyce HW Jr, Brown JI, et al. A new objective measurement of esophageal lumen patency. Am J Gastroenterol 1989;84:1255–8.
41. Lipka S, Keshishian J, Boyce HW, et al. The natural history of steroid-naïve eosinophilic esophagitis in adults treated with endoscopic dilation and PPIs over a mean duration of nearly 14 years. Gastrointest Endosc 2014;80:592–8.
42. Lipka S, Kumar A, Richter JE. Esophageal remodeling in eosinophilic esophagitis patients undergoing dilation over a mean 10 year follow-up. Gastroenterology 2015;148:S794–5.
43. Madanick RD, Shaheen NJ, Dellon ES. A novel balloon pull-through technique for esophageal dilation in eosinophilic esophagitis. Gastrointest Endosc 2011;73:138–42.
44. Robles-Medranda C, Villard F, LeGall C, et al. Severe dysphagia in children with eosinophilic esophagitis and esophageal stricture: an indication for balloon dilation? J Pediatr Gastroenterol Nutr 2010;50:516–20.
45. Menard-Kutcher C, Furuta GT, Kramer RE. Dilation of pediatric eosinophilic esophagitis – adverse events and short term outcome. J Pediatr Gastroenterol Nutr 2017;64(5):701–6.
46. Lipka S, Kumar A, Richter JE. Successful esophageal dilation of eosinophilic esophagitis patients with previous post-dilation complications: start low and go slow. J Clin Gastroenterol 2017. [Epub ahead of print].

# Future Directions in Eosinophilic Esophagitis

Ikuo Hirano, MD

## KEYWORDS

- Eosinophilic esophagitis • Gastroesophageal reflux disease • Dysphagia
- Food allergy • Esophageal stricture • Esophagitis

## KEY POINTS

- Advances in awareness, scientific understanding, and treatment options for eosinophilic esophagitis have paralleled the dramatic increase in the prevalence of this relatively newly identified esophageal disorder.
- Future directions include efforts to refine the diagnostic criteria, identify genetic and environmental risk factors, appreciate the contribution of inflammatory pathways and cellular elements beyond the eosinophil, recognize the importance of subepithelial remodeling, validate appropriate endpoints for therapeutic trials, define a role for targeted biologic therapies, and optimize approaches to dietary therapy.
- From the perspective of gastrointestinal endoscopy, endoscopic outcomes have emerged as an objective and reproducible endpoint in clinical trials of novel therapeutics in eosinophilic esophagitis that complement current activity measures of symptoms and histology.
- Ongoing efforts continue to develop novel, less invasive methods to assess the activity of eosinophic esophagitis to obviate the need for repeated endoscopy.
- Assessment of esophageal distensibility using the functional lumen imaging probe have demonstrated clinical relevance as an important determinant of disease complications and potential utility as a therapeutic endpoint in eosinophilic esophagitis.

Over the past 2 decades, tremendous progress has been made in understanding the diagnosis, epidemiology, pathogenesis, and treatment of eosinophilic esophagitis (EoE).[1] At the same time, major questions and controversies have arisen. The diagnostic criteria, reasons for the growing incidence, appropriate therapeutic endpoints, and efficacy of nonsteroid therapeutic options are among these. This article summarizes and speculates on future issues facing both clinicians and investigators entering the third decade of EoE.

Disclosures: Ikuo Hirano Consulting: Adare, Celgene, Regeneron, Shire. Research funding: Celgene, Regeneron, Shire.
Division of Gastroenterology, Northwestern University Feinberg School of Medicine, 676 North Saint Clair, Suite 1400, Chicago, IL 60611, USA

## DIAGNOSIS: BEYOND THE EOSINOPHIL

The diagnosis of EoE combines clinical manifestations of esophageal dysfunction with esophageal histopathologic features of eosinophil predominant inflammation.[2] Before the recognition of EoE, eosinophil-predominant inflammation was considered a hallmark of gastroesophageal reflux disease (GERD). To distinguish EoE from GERD, a therapeutic trial of proton pump inhibitor (PPI) therapy was recommended as a means of excluding GERD based on the persistence of eosinophilia.[3] Recent studies have noted that patients with esophageal eosinophilia that resolves with PPI therapy, or PPI-responsive esophageal eosinophilia (PPIREE), are demographically, symptomatically, endoscopically, histologically, and genetically largely identical to EoE.[4,5] Thus, emerging consensus recommendations have advocated that the PPI trial be removed from the diagnostic criteria for EoE.[5] Instead, the contribution of disorders that may resemble, cause, or contribute to the clinical presentation of EoE (eg, GERD, lichen planus, radiation esophagitis, graft-versus-host disease) and histologic manifestations (eg, GERD, Crohn disease, drug hypersensitivity) are considered before a formal diagnosis of EoE, without mandating a formal PPI trial. As the operational definition of EoE evolves, challenges in the near-term include clarifying whether the similar baseline characteristics between EoE and PPIREE translate to equivalent response to specific therapeutic interventions (ie, do patients with EoE and PPIREE have similar response rates to either diet or steroids).[6,7] The significance of this distinction affects the generalizability of the existing literature on EoE therapy that has predominantly focused on the subset of patients who have not responded to PPI. The mechanisms responsible for the reported 25% to 50% histologic response to PPI therapy need elucidation regarding the relative importance of acid suppression and recently identified, anti-inflammatory properties of PPI therapy.[8–10] Future studies examining the complex interactions between acid reflux, PPI therapy, and antigen-triggered immune responses will improve understanding of both the pathogenesis and treatment of EoE.

Molecular and genetic characterization of EoE continues to advance the understanding of the pathogenesis and has identified novel biomarkers that characterize the disease.[11] Recently, a cohort of 5 adult subjects with dysphagia of unclear cause responsive to corticosteroids but without esophageal eosinophils was described.[12] These subjects had increased T-lymphocytes in the esophageal epithelium compared with controls. Messenger RNA tissue expression of certain genes (MUC4, CDH26) upregulated in EoE were observed but did not include eotaxin-3 expression. This novel observation suggests that EoE may represent a part of a larger, chronic, esophageal inflammatory disease involving T-lymphocytes. Although less common than EoE, increasing reports of patients with dysphagia and endoscopic features of EoE with numerous esophageal intraepithelial lymphocytes without eosinophilia have been characterized as lymphocytic esophagitis (**Fig. 1**). It remains unclear if these patients are a distinct entity or part of an evolving spectrum that includes EoE. Several studies have identified a distinct mast cell signature in the esophageal epithelium of both children and adults with EoE.[13–16] In another study, the role of basophils in the pathogenesis of EoE was demonstrated in a murine model.[17] Depletion of basophils in a novel, ovalbumin-sensitized murine model of EoE led to significant reduction in esophageal eosinophilia and expression of type 2 T helper cell cytokine response. These important studies open the door to the exploration of the role of inflammatory cells beyond the eosinophil in disease pathogenesis and utility of novel biomarkers in the definition of EoE. The importance of these elements is being explored with therapeutics that target specific cell types.

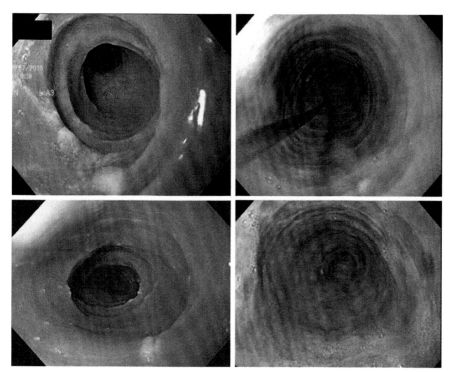

**Fig. 1.** Endoscopic images from a patient with lymphocytic esophagitis. Endoscopic features of loss of vascular markings, ring-like strictures, and exudate mimic the typical appearance of EoE. Biopsies over a 3-year span showed persistent marked lymphocytic infiltration of the esophageal mucosa without eosinophilia. The patient had no evidence of reflux esophagitis or lichen planus.

Future directions in the diagnosis and understanding of EoE may move away from the existing diagnostic criteria of EoE that are based on clinical and pathologic parameters. Limitations to the current definition include the exclusion of patients with preclinical disease (ie, esophageal eosinophilia in the absence of symptoms despite endoscopic or molecular features) and patients with incomplete expression of predetermined biological parameters (ie, patients with clinical and endoscopic manifestations of EoE but <15 eosinophils per high-power field). As previously mentioned, recent research has uncovered potentially important roles for T-lymphocytes, basophils, and mast cells that are not included in current diagnostic criteria. A systems approach to medical disease incorporates complex interactions between clinical phenotypes, genetics, environmental factors, and intermediate phenotypes that may provide a more accurate representation of disease and direct a more personalized approach to management.[18] A proposed example of a modular network for EoE is shown in **Fig. 2**. Future studies could define probabilistic relationships between the elements to identify regulatory nodes that modify phenotypes. For instance, patients with a phenotype favoring the development of fibrostenosis would be considered for therapies targeting remodeling pathways. Other patients with predefined clinical, genetic, and environmental signatures signifying a low risk for disease progression may not warrant therapeutic intervention.

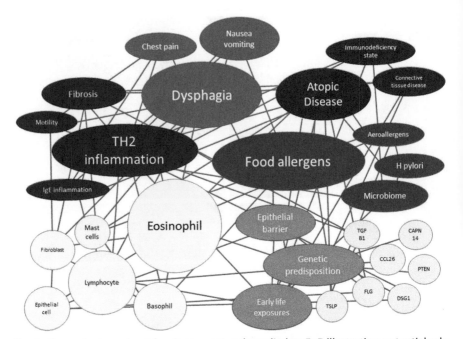

**Fig. 2.** Conceptual construct for disease network applied to EoE illustrating potential relationships among clinical, genetic, environmental, and immunologic determinants of pathophenotypes. With future studies, probabilistic weighting of the relative importance of distinct nodes in the network, as well as the strength of relationships between notes, are assigned to provide a more complex but also more accurate depiction of EoE. Key: blue clinical phenotypes; green, environmental determinants; orange, genetic determinants; purple, disease-modifying host factors; red intermediate phenotypes; yellow, cellular elements.

## EPIDEMIOLOGY: BEYOND AN ORPHAN DISEASE

Current incidence estimates for EoE vary from 5 to 10 cases per 100,000 with prevalence estimates on the order of 0.5 to 1 case per 1000. Studies have also demonstrated a dramatic increase in the incidence of EoE over the past 2 decades, even when accounting for the increased utilization of upper endoscopy.[19] Based on the steady increase, it is projected that EoE will soon surpass the threshold for orphan disease designation (200,000 in the United States).

The high prevalence of EoE in Western countries compared with Eastern and sub-Saharan countries provides an opportunity to investigate the influence of racial, genetic, and environmental factors that contribute to the development of disease. Ongoing and future identification of risk factors contributing to the emergence of EoE should provide invaluable insights into the underlying cause of EoE. Studies of early life exposures have identified antibiotic exposure during the first year of life, breast feeding, Cesarean delivery, and preterm birth with increased risk of EoE.[20] Although genetic risk variants have been identified, a study examining inherited risks among twins and siblings of affected patients with EoE demonstrated that most family clustering of EoE was attributable to environmental rather than genetic factors.[20]

Alterations in the gut microbiome over the past few decades have been proposed as a contributing factor for the emergence of EoE. Murine models have demonstrated the impact of alternations in the gut microbiome in the risk for development of asthma and colitis.[21] Marked effects of diet on the microbiome are of particular interest given the established relationship between diet and the pathogenesis of EoE. Two groups have reported alterations in the esophageal microbiome of patients with active EoE.[22,23] Additional infectious risk factors for EoE have been reported. Multiple studies from around the world have shown an inverse association between *Helicobacter pylori* and EoE.[24–26] This association is noteworthy given the widespread treatment of *H pylori* over the past 3 decades, as well as prior studies noting a similar inverse association with asthma, allergic rhinitis, and atopic dermatitis. It is also possible that the presence of *H pylori* is a surrogate marker of the hygiene status of an at-risk population and not directly involved in the pathogenesis of EoE. Recently, administration of a specific strain of *Lactobacillus* led to significant improvement in esophageal eosinophilia in a murine model of EoE.[27] Future studies examining the role of *H pylori*, as well as the esophageal microbiome, will further address these important observations that have profound implications for both disease origin and novel treatment approaches.

## EVALUATION: BEYOND THE ESOPHAGEAL MUCOSA

The primary complications of EoE arise as a consequence of esophageal remodeling in the setting of chronic inflammation.[28] Manifestations of dysphagia and food impaction are directly related to esophageal luminal compromise. Esophageal perforation in EoE typically occurs in the setting of food impaction or esophageal dilation and thus are also the result of remodeling. In addition, the transmural involvement of both inflammation and fibrosis may contribute to an increased risk of esophageal rupture.[28–30] The most consistently identified predictor of risk of stenosis in EoE is duration of disease. In a retrospective study, more than 60% of subjects with disease duration of more than 10 years had clinically significant esophageal strictures.[31] Esophageal epithelial mesenchymal transition and subepithelial fibrosis are integral to the remodeling process.[32] Detection of subepithelial fibrosis on esophageal biopsy has been reported as a common finding in both pediatric and adult EoE.[33,34] However, standard biopsy forceps assess the subepithelial space in the minority of cases. Moreover, the correlation between the severity of collagen deposition on biopsies and the severity of esophageal strictures has not been demonstrated, limiting the utility of the quantification of lamina propria fibrosis outside of research settings. Additional studies using endoluminal ultrasonography have confirmed the presence of subepithelial esophageal remodeling with significant expansion of the mucosa, submucosa, and muscularis propria in EoE.[35]

In clinical practice, esophageal remodeling is primarily assessed by means of barium esophagram or upper endoscopy. Although barium studies can assess normal patency of the esophageal lumen, the accuracy of stricture severity is limited by the inability to control for intraluminal pressure with a swallowed bolus. Radiation exposure and the need to have a separate test by radiology are other drawbacks. Endoscopic assessment of strictures is readily available because endoscopy is routinely performed in EoE for purposes of biopsy acquisition. However, the accuracy of endoscopy assessment is also limited, with overall low sensitivity for stricture detection.[36] The severity of esophageal ring formation based on the EoE Endoscopic Reference Score (EREFS) correlates with the degree of overall luminal restriction but provides an imprecise measure of remodeling.[37,38]

The consequence of esophageal remodeling can be demonstrated in patients during endoscopy using the functional luminal imaging probe (FLIP, Crospon, Ireland). This catheter-based technique provides quantitative readouts regarding the physical properties of the esophageal wall, including contractile activity and mural distensibility.[39] Significant reduction in esophageal distensibility has been demonstrated in both children and adults with EoE.[40,41] Moreover, measurements of esophageal distensibility have been shown to correlate with clinically relevant outcomes of food impaction in EoE.[40,42] Given intrinsic limitations in symptom assessment as a primary endpoint in EoE (ie, careful mastication or food avoidance can circumvent detection of dysphagia symptoms) and histology (dysphagia is more closely linked to subepithelial remodeling than mucosal eosinophilia), distensibility offers a clinically relevant and quantitative assessment of disease activity.[43] Thus, current applications of FLIP technology are examining its utility as a biomarker for remodeling in the context of clinical trials of novel therapeutics in EoE. A small, proof-of-concept study has demonstrated the capability of FLIP to detect clinically meaningful improvements in esophageal distensibility using topical steroids or elimination diet therapy.[44] A future direction in FLIP analyses is depicting data with graphical depiction of multiple foci of the esophagus rather than with current metrics that limit the analysis to a single point of minimum esophageal distensibility. Real-time, topographic, color contour plots are able to depict regional variation in esophageal distensibility along the axial length of the esophagus (**Fig. 3**).[39,45] With this graphical depiction, more global improvement in esophageal remodeling after therapeutic intervention becomes readily apparent.

## TREATMENT ENDPOINTS: BEYOND COUNTING EOSINOPHILS

Advances in medical therapy for EoE rely on the use of clinically relevant and validated endpoints that assess disease activity and are responsive to intervention.

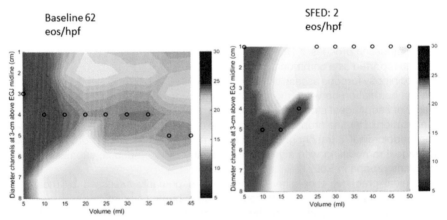

**Fig. 3.** Color topographic depiction of a FLIP distension study of an adult patient with EoE before and after 6-food elimination diet therapy. The plots depict esophageal luminal diameter across multiple longitudinal locations (Y-axis) during volumetric distension of the lumen up to 45 to 50 mL using a 16-cm balloon catheter (X-axis). Color represents luminal diameters with warm colors (*red*) depicting small diameters and cold colors (*blue*) depicting large diameters. Before treatment (*left panel*), the patient has active inflammation with 62 eosinophils per high-power field (hpf) on biopsy. The FLIP plot clearly demonstrated reduced distensibility of most the interrogated esophagus, with luminal diameters of less than 14 mm. Following treatment, there is a marked improvement in esophageal inflammation with biopsies showing a peak eosinophil density of 2 eosinophils per hpf. Corresponding with this histologic response, the FLIP plot (*right panel*) depicts and improvement in distensibility with diameters exceeding 17 mm. eos, eosinophils; EGJ, esophagogastric junction.

Currently, improvement in the coprimary endpoints of symptoms and esophageal eosinophilia define success of therapeutics in EoE.[43] Unfortunately, both outcomes have serious limitations. Symptoms can be quite sporadic, even for patients with severe disease, due to adaptive eating behaviors such as meticulous mastication, prolonged meal times, and food avoidance. The Eosinophilic Esophagitis Activity Index (EEsAI) was developed to provide a patient-reported outcome instrument that accounts for such adaptive behaviors and is now being tested for responsiveness in clinical trials.[46] Another drawback to reliance on symptom outcomes is that symptoms reflect a combination of esophageal remodeling and, to a lesser degree, inflammatory activity. Thus, basing the success of a medication that targets inflammation on symptom improvement may underestimate the anti-inflammatory benefits. A clear example of this discordance is the marked symptom improvement following esophageal dilation that can occur without altering mucosal eosinophilia.

Currently, eosinophil density is a primary outcome determinant of inflammatory activity in EoE. The metric is well-positioned as a therapeutic endpoint given the high degree of interobserver and intraobserver reliability, and widespread acceptance as a defining and objective feature of EoE. However, eosinophil density has shown limited correlation with either symptom or endoscopic activity. The recently described Histology Scoring System (HSS) provides a more comprehensive assessment of esophageal disease that includes tissue injury patterns and assessment of both the severity (grade) and extent (stage) of histologic activity.[47] Further validation of the responsiveness of the HSS in the context of clinical trials is ongoing.

Endoscopic outcomes have conceptual advantages of providing a whole organ view that includes both inflammatory and remodeling aspects. The EREFS has been validated and already demonstrated responsiveness as a secondary endpoint in clinical trials.[38] Improvement in endoscopic appearance supports evidence of symptom and histologic improvement. Future studies are optimizing the scoring of individual features of the EREFS to increase the performance of the instrument. Other novel biomarkers of disease being looked at as endpoints in clinical trials include the EoE Diagnostic Panel that provides data on genetic expression and the FLIP measures of esophageal distensibility previously discussed.

## MEDICAL THERAPY: BEYOND TOPICAL CORTICOSTEROIDS

Short-term future directions in the medical therapy for EoE include review and approval by regulatory authorities of novel formulations of topical corticosteroids that are optimized for esophageal delivery. The current practice of having patients swallow the aerosolized mist from a metered-dose inhaler designed for asthma is clearly suboptimal. In addition, concerns for the systemic absorption of steroids that are being dosed at 2 to 10 times the doses used for allergic rhinitis and asthma have raised concerns regarding the risk for adrenal suppression, cataracts, and growth suppression in children. Moreover, although highly efficacious, topical steroids have demonstrated histologic response rates that vary from 40% to 90%, leading to a large group of steroid-nonresponders.[48]

Longer term directions in EoE therapy include examining the potential benefits of biologic therapies. Biologic or immunomodulator therapy offer therapeutic options for steroid refractory patients. Therapies targeting specific allergic pathways offer putative advantages for EoE patients, most of whom have multiple forms of atopy, including asthma, allergic rhinitis, food allergy mediated by immunoglobulin (Ig)-E, and atopic dermatitis. Systemic therapy targeting remodeling pathways may prevent or reverse existing fibrostenosis, as well as arrest inflammation. On a practical level, long duration responses to systemic therapies offer practical advantages of intermittent therapy compared with the daily administration of topical steroids. Several antibody therapies have already demonstrated efficacy in randomized controlled trials. Anti-interleukin (IL)-5 therapy using mepolizumab and reslizumab demonstrated significant reductions in esophageal mucosal eosinophilia compared with controls in 3 randomized controlled trials.[49–51] Antibodies targeting IL-13 delivered via a weekly subcutaneous injection demonstrated substantial reductions in esophageal eosinophilia, as well as improvement in symptoms, particularly in steroid refractory patients.[52,53]

## DIET THERAPY: BEYOND 6-FOOD ELIMINATION DIET PROTOCOL

Diet therapy was the first therapy described for the treatment of EoE and has remained an important and highly effective treatment option. It is an attractive alternative from the patient's perspective, offering a nonpharmacologic alternative for maintenance of disease remission.[54] The biggest drawback of diet therapy is the need for repeated endoscopies during food reintroduction to allow for detection of specific food triggers. This protocol can necessitate 5 to 10 endoscopic procedures, depending on the number of food groups that were initially removed during the induction phase of treatment. Future directions in diet therapy are thus focused on reducing the number of endoscopic procedures required for identification of food triggers for an individual patient. Current strategies have relied on the 6-food elimination diet protocol but newer protocols are examining the use of 1-, 2-, and 4-food approaches that limit the induction phase food elimination to the most likely food triggers (ie, milk, wheat, egg, soy).[55–58] Practical problems with this streamlined approach are an anticipated lower response to the induction phase, as well as potential for missing combination of food triggers. Also undergoing validation are approaches that allow for less invasive or less costly detection of EoE disease activity. Transnasal endoscopy using ultrathin endoscopes acquires esophageal biopsies without anesthesia, thereby limiting cost.[59,60] Two novel technologies involve ingestion of dissolving capsules that deploy a string or sponge to sample esophageal contents. The esophageal string test (Enterotrack, Aurora Colorado) measures eosinophil based proteins in luminal secretions that adhere to the string while positioned in the esophagus.[61] Initial studies have reported accuracy for differentiating active from inactive EoE. The cytosponge was designed to perform cytologic analyses of Barrett's esophagus. Application to EoE has demonstrated good test performance compared with the gold standard of esophageal biopsy.[62]

Future approaches to diet therapy will move beyond the elimination–reintroduction approach and focus on accurate in vitro, in vivo, or serologic tests to identify trigger foods. Detection of expressed biomarkers in tissue biopsies or cultured esophageal epithelial cells following exposure to food antigens may offer a bioassay to assess for food triggers. Recent interest in increased food-specific IgG4 expression has sparked studies looking at the potential predictive value of this assessment for diet triggers in EoE.[63] A preliminary, small study performed injection of several suspected food extracts into the esophageal submucosa during endoscopy.[64] An acute and pronounced esophageal contraction, as well as delayed, wheal-type mucosal reaction at the site of food inoculation were detected. The investigators hope that this type of protocol may allow for immediate identification of causative foods in EoE. Understanding the underlying pathogenesis of EoE in the context of the dramatic increase in atopy will undoubtedly reveal novel therapeutic approaches.

## SUMMARY

Advances in the awareness, scientific understanding, and treatment options for EoE have paralleled the dramatic increase in the prevalence of this relatively newly identified esophageal disorder. Future directions include efforts to refine the diagnostic criteria, identify genetic and environmental risk factors, appreciate the contribution of inflammatory pathways and cellular elements beyond the eosinophil, recognize the importance of subepithelial remodeling, validate appropriate endpoints for therapeutic trials, and optimize approaches to dietary therapy. Although tremendous progress has been made over the past 2 decades since the initial descriptions of EoE, areas of uncertainty and controversy continue to challenge clinicians and investigators from multiple specialties who have the common goal of improving patient care.

## REFERENCES

1. Hirano I. 2015 David Y. Graham Lecture: the first two decades of eosinophilic esophagitis-from acid reflux to food allergy. Am J Gastroenterol 2016;111(6): 770–6.
2. Liacouras CA, Furuta GT, Hirano I, et al. Eosinophilic esophagitis: updated consensus recommendations for children and adults. J Allergy Clin Immunol 2011;128(1):3–20.e6 [quiz: 1–2].
3. Furuta GT, Liacouras CA, Collins MH, et al. Eosinophilic esophagitis in children and adults: a systematic review and consensus recommendations for diagnosis and treatment. Gastroenterology 2007;133(4):1342–63.
4. Kia L, Hirano I. Distinguishing GERD from eosinophilic oesophagitis: concepts and controversies. Nat Rev Gastroenterol Hepatol 2015;12(7):379–86.
5. Molina-Infante J, Bredenoord AJ, Cheng E, et al. Proton pump inhibitor-responsive oesophageal eosinophilia: an entity challenging current diagnostic criteria for eosinophilic oesophagitis. Gut 2016;65(3):524–31.
6. Sodikoff J, Hirano I. Proton pump inhibitor-responsive esophageal eosinophilia does not preclude food-responsive eosinophilic esophagitis. J Allergy Clin Immunol 2016;137(2):631–3.
7. Lucendo AJ, Arias A, Gonzalez-Cervera J, et al. Dual response to dietary/topical steroid and proton pump inhibitor therapy in adult patients with eosinophilic esophagitis. J Allergy Clin Immunol 2016;137(3):931–4.e2.
8. Cheng E, Souza RF, Spechler SJ. Eosinophilic esophagitis: interactions with gastroesophageal reflux disease. Gastroenterol Clin North Am 2014;43(2): 243–56.
9. Cheng E, Zhang X, Huo X, et al. Omeprazole blocks eotaxin-3 expression by oesophageal squamous cells from patients with eosinophilic oesophagitis and GORD. Gut 2013;62(6):824–32.
10. Spechler SJ, Genta RM, Souza RF. Thoughts on the complex relationship between gastroesophageal reflux disease and eosinophilic esophagitis. Am J Gastroenterol 2007;102(6):1301–6.
11. Rothenberg ME. Molecular, genetic, and cellular bases for treating eosinophilic esophagitis. Gastroenterology 2015;148(6):1143–57.
12. Straumann A, Blanchard C, Radonjic-Hoesli S, et al. A new eosinophilic esophagitis (EoE)-like disease without tissue eosinophilia found in EoE families. Allergy 2016;71(6):889–900.
13. Aceves SS, Chen D, Newbury RO, et al. Mast cells infiltrate the esophageal smooth muscle in patients with eosinophilic esophagitis, express TGF-beta1,

and increase esophageal smooth muscle contraction. J Allergy Clin Immunol 2010;126(6):1198–204.e4.

14. Abonia JP, Blanchard C, Butz BB, et al. Involvement of mast cells in eosinophilic esophagitis. J Allergy Clin Immunol 2010;126(1):140–9.

15. Hsu Blatman KS, Gonsalves N, Hirano I, et al. Expression of mast cell-associated genes is upregulated in adult eosinophilic esophagitis and responds to steroid or dietary therapy. J Allergy Clin Immunol 2011;127(5):1307–8.e3.

16. Dellon ES, Chen X, Miller CR, et al. Tryptase staining of mast cells may differentiate eosinophilic esophagitis from gastroesophageal reflux disease. Am J Gastroenterol 2011;106(2):264–71.

17. Noti M, Wojno ED, Kim BS, et al. Thymic stromal lymphopoietin-elicited basophil responses promote eosinophilic esophagitis. Nat Med 2013;19(8):1005–13.

18. Loscalzo J, Kohane I, Barabasi AL. Human disease classification in the postgenomic era: a complex systems approach to human pathobiology. Mol Syst Biol 2007;3:124.

19. Dellon ES. Epidemiology of eosinophilic esophagitis. Gastroenterol Clin North Am 2014;43(2):201–18.

20. Alexander ES, Martin LJ, Collins MH, et al. Twin and family studies reveal strong environmental and weaker genetic cues explaining heritability of eosinophilic esophagitis. J Allergy Clin Immunol 2014;134(5):1084–92.e1.

21. Honda K, Littman DR. The microbiota in adaptive immune homeostasis and disease. Nature 2016;535(7610):75–84.

22. Harris JK, Fang R, Wagner BD, et al. Esophageal microbiome in eosinophilic esophagitis. PLoS One 2015;10(5):e0128346.

23. Benitez AJ, Hoffmann C, Muir AB, et al. Inflammation-associated microbiota in pediatric eosinophilic esophagitis. Microbiome 2015;3:23.

24. Dellon ES, Peery AF, Shaheen NJ, et al. Inverse association of esophageal eosinophilia with *Helicobacter pylori* based on analysis of a US pathology database. Gastroenterology 2011;141(5):1586–92.

25. von Arnim U, Wex T, Link A, et al. *Helicobacter pylori* infection is associated with a reduced risk of developing eosinophilic oesophagitis. Aliment Pharmacol Ther 2016;43(7):825–30.

26. Sonnenberg A, Dellon ES, Turner KO, et al. The influence of *Helicobacter pylori* on the ethnic distribution of esophageal eosinophilia. Helicobacter 2017;22(3). http://dx.doi.org/10.1111/hel.12370.

27. Holvoet S, Doucet-Ladeveze R, Perrot M, et al. Beneficial effect of *Lactococcus lactis* NCC 2287 in a murine model of eosinophilic esophagitis. Allergy 2016; 71(12):1753–61.

28. Hirano I, Aceves SS. Clinical implications and pathogenesis of esophageal remodeling in eosinophilic esophagitis. Gastroenterol Clin North Am 2014;43(2): 297–316.

29. Straumann A, Rossi L, Simon HU, et al. Fragility of the esophageal mucosa: a pathognomonic endoscopic sign of primary eosinophilic esophagitis? Gastrointest Endosc 2003;57(3):407–12.

30. Rieder F, Nonevski I, Ma J, et al. T-helper 2 cytokines, transforming growth factor beta1, and eosinophil products induce fibrogenesis and alter muscle motility in patients with eosinophilic esophagitis. Gastroenterology 2014;146(5): 1266–77.e1-9.

31. Schoepfer AM, Safroneeva E, Bussmann C, et al. Delay in diagnosis of eosinophilic esophagitis increases risk for stricture formation in a time-dependent manner. Gastroenterology 2013;145(6):1230–6.e1-2.

32. Kagalwalla AF, Akhtar N, Woodruff SA, et al. Eosinophilic esophagitis: epithelial mesenchymal transition contributes to esophageal remodeling and reverses with treatment. J Allergy Clin Immunol 2012;129(5):1387–96.e7.

33. Aceves SS, Newbury RO, Dohil R, et al. Esophageal remodeling in pediatric eosinophilic esophagitis. J Allergy Clin Immunol 2007;119(1):206–12.

34. Aceves SS, Newbury RO, Chen D, et al. Resolution of remodeling in eosinophilic esophagitis correlates with epithelial response to topical corticosteroids. Allergy 2010;65(1):109–16.

35. Straumann A, Conus S, Degen L, et al. Long-term budesonide maintenance treatment is partially effective for patients with eosinophilic esophagitis. Clin Gastroenterol Hepatol 2011;9(5):400–9.e1.

36. Gentile N, Katzka D, Ravi K, et al. Oesophageal narrowing is common and frequently under-appreciated at endoscopy in patients with oesophageal eosinophilia. Aliment Pharmacol Ther 2014;40(11–12):1333–40.

37. Chen JW, Pandolfino JE, Lin Z, et al. Severity of endoscopically identified esophageal rings correlates with reduced esophageal distensibility in eosinophilic esophagitis. Endoscopy 2016;48(9):794–801.

38. Hirano I, Moy N, Heckman MG, et al. Endoscopic assessment of the oesophageal features of eosinophilic oesophagitis: validation of a novel classification and grading system. Gut 2013;62(4):489–95.

39. Hirano I, Pandolfino JE, Boeckxstaens GE. Functional lumen imaging probe for the management of esophageal disorders: expert review from the clinical practice updates committee of the AGA Institute. Clin Gastroenterol Hepatol 2017; 15(3):325–34.

40. Menard-Katcher C, Benitez AJ, Pan Z, et al. Influence of age and eosinophilic esophagitis on esophageal distensibility in a pediatric cohort. Am J Gastroenterol 2017. [Epub ahead of print].

41. Kwiatek MA, Hirano I, Kahrilas PJ, et al. Mechanical properties of the esophagus in eosinophilic esophagitis. Gastroenterology 2011;140(1):82–90, epub ahead of print.

42. Nicodeme F, Hirano I, Chen J, et al. Esophageal distensibility as a measure of disease severity in patients with eosinophilic esophagitis. Clin Gastroenterol Hepatol 2013;11(9):1101–7.e1.

43. Hirano I, Spechler S, Furuta G, et al. White paper AGA: eosinophilic esophagitis. Clin Gastroenterol Hepatol 2017;15(8):1173–83.

44. Carlson DA, Hirano I, Zalewski A, et al. Changes in esophageal distensibility associated with treatment response in eosinophilic esophagitis: a study utilizing the functional lumen imaging probe. Gastroenterology 2017;152(5):S108.

45. Lin Z, Kahrilas PJ, Xiao Y, et al. Functional luminal imaging probe topography: an improved method for characterizing esophageal distensibility in eosinophilic esophagitis. Ther Adv Gastroenterol 2013;6(2):97–107.

46. Schoepfer AM, Straumann A, Panczak R, et al. Development and validation of a symptom-based activity index for adults with eosinophilic esophagitis. Gastroenterology 2014;147(6):1255–66.e21.

47. Collins MH, Martin LJ, Alexander ES, et al. Newly developed and validated eosinophilic esophagitis histology scoring system and evidence that it outperforms peak eosinophil count for disease diagnosis and monitoring. Dis Esophagus 2017;30(3):1–8.

48. Kavitt RT, Hirano I, Vaezi MF. Diagnosis and treatment of eosinophilic esophagitis in adults. Am J Med 2016;129(9):924–34.

49. Assa'ad AH, Gupta SK, Collins MH, et al. An antibody against IL-5 reduces numbers of esophageal intraepithelial eosinophils in children with eosinophilic esophagitis. Gastroenterology 2011;141(5):1593–604.

50. Spergel JM, Rothenberg ME, Collins MH, et al. Reslizumab in children and adolescents with eosinophilic esophagitis: results of a double-blind, randomized, placebo-controlled trial. J Allergy Clin Immunol 2012;129(2):456–63, 63.e1–3.

51. Straumann A, Conus S, Grzonka P, et al. Anti-interleukin-5 antibody treatment (mepolizumab) in active eosinophilic oesophagitis: a randomised, placebo-controlled, double-blind trial. Gut 2010;59(1):21–30.

52. Rothenberg ME, Wen T, Greenberg A, et al. Intravenous anti-IL-13 mAb QAX576 for the treatment of eosinophilic esophagitis. J Allergy Clin Immunol 2015;135(2):500–7.

53. Hirano I, Collins MH, Assouline-Dayan Y, et al. A randomized, double-blind, placebo-controlled trial of a novel recombinant, humanized, anti-interleukin-13 monoclonal antibody (RPC4046) in patients with active eosinophilic esophagitis: results of the HEROES study. United Eur Gastroenterol J 2016.

54. Doerfler B, Bryce P, Hirano I, et al. Practical approach to implementing dietary therapy in adults with eosinophilic esophagitis: the Chicago experience. Dis Esophagus 2015;28(1):42–58.

55. Gonsalves N, Yang GY, Doerfler B, et al. Elimination diet effectively treats eosinophilic esophagitis in adults; food reintroduction identifies causative factors. Gastroenterology 2012;142(7):1451–9.e1 [quiz: e14–5].

56. Lucendo AJ, Arias A, Gonzalez-Cervera J, et al. Empiric 6-food elimination diet induced and maintained prolonged remission in patients with adult eosinophilic esophagitis: a prospective study on the food cause of the disease. J Allergy Clin Immunol 2013;131(3):797–804.

57. Molina-Infante J, Arias A, Barrio J, et al. Four-food group elimination diet for adult eosinophilic esophagitis: a prospective multicenter study. J Allergy Clin Immunol 2014;134(5):1093–9.e1.

58. Kagalwalla AF, Amsden K, Shah A, et al. Cow's milk elimination: a novel dietary approach to treat eosinophilic esophagitis. J Pediatr Gastroenterol Nutr 2012;55(6):711–6.

59. Friedlander JA, DeBoer EM, Soden JS, et al. Unsedated transnasal esophagoscopy for monitoring therapy in pediatric eosinophilic esophagitis. Gastrointest Endosc 2016;83(2):299–306.e1.

60. Philpott H, Nandurkar S, Royce SG, et al. Ultrathin unsedated transnasal gastroscopy in monitoring eosinophilic esophagitis. J Gastroenterol Hepatol 2016;31(3):590–4.

61. Furuta GT, Kagalwalla AF, Lee JJ, et al. The oesophageal string test: a novel, minimally invasive method measures mucosal inflammation in eosinophilic oesophagitis. Gut 2013;62(10):1395–405.

62. Katzka DA, Geno DM, Ravi A, et al. Accuracy, safety, and tolerability of tissue collection by Cytosponge vs endoscopy for evaluation of eosinophilic esophagitis. Clin Gastroenterol Hepatol 2015;13(1):77–83.e2.

63. Clayton F, Fang JC, Gleich GJ, et al. Eosinophilic esophagitis in adults is associated with IgG4 and not mediated by IgE. Gastroenterology 2014;147(3):602–9.

64. Warners MJ, Terreehorst I, van den Wijngaard RM, et al. Development of a new diagnostic test for esophageal food sensitization in adult EOE patients: the Gastroscopic Esophageal Prick Test (EPT). Gastroenterology 2017;152(5):S165.

# Moving?

## Make sure your subscription moves with you!

To notify us of your new address, find your **Clinics Account Number** (located on your mailing label above your name), and contact customer service at:

**Email: journalscustomerservice-usa@elsevier.com**

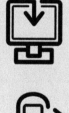

**800-654-2452** (subscribers in the U.S. & Canada)
**314-447-8871** (subscribers outside of the U.S. & Canada)

**Fax number: 314-447-8029**

**Elsevier Health Sciences Division**
**Subscription Customer Service**
**3251 Riverport Lane**
**Maryland Heights, MO 63043**

*To ensure uninterrupted delivery of your subscription, please notify us at least 4 weeks in advance of move.

Printed and bound by CPI Group (UK) Ltd, Croydon, CR0 4YY

08/05/2025

01864703-0006